RETHINKING DIABETES

RETHINKING DIABETES

*Entanglements with Trauma,
Poverty, and HIV*

EMILY MENDENHALL

Foreword by Mark Nichter

CORNELL UNIVERSITY PRESS
ITHACA AND LONDON

First published 2019 by Cornell University Press

Library of Congress Cataloging-in-Publication Data

Names: Mendenhall, Emily, 1982– author.
Title: Rethinking diabetes : entanglements with poverty, trauma,
    and HIV / Emily Mendenhall.
Description: Ithaca [New York] : Cornell University Press, 2019. |
    Includes bibliographical references and index.
Identifiers: LCCN 2018052012 (print) | LCCN 2018052992 (ebook) |
    ISBN 9781501738319 (pdf) | ISBN 9781501738326 (ret) |
    ISBN 9781501738302 | ISBN 9781501738302 (cloth) |
    ISBN 9781501738432 (pbk.)
Subjects: LCSH: Diabetes—Social aspects. | Diabetes—Economic
    aspects. | Diabetes—Psychosomatic aspects. | Diabetes—Psychological
    aspects. | Diabetes in women. | Diabetics—Social conditions—
    21st century. | Syndemics.
Classification: LCC RA645.D5 (ebook) |
    LCC RA645.D5 M458 2019 (print) | DDC 362.1964/62—dc23
LC record available at https://lccn.loc.gov/2018052012

For Adam,
in thanks for everything you did to support me
in writing this book

CONTENTS

FOREWORD

Mark Nichter

One of my key informants in South India between the mid 1970s and late 1990s was an ayurvedic practitioner (*vaidya*) who had also received integrated medicine training from a medical college in Madras. He was renowned for the treatment of diabetes and was referred patients by both allopathic and ayurvedic practitioners. In the 1970s I watched him treat a steady stream of patients from all walks of life. Most had already been diagnosed with diabetes and had seen several practitioners. Patients typically brought with them the results of lab tests and bags of medications prescribed by other practitioners. I carefully observed his interactions with patients and was struck by the way he treated patients having the same allopathic diagnosis with different types of medicine and dietary advice.

The vaidya observed my interest in his treatment of diabetes and used it as an opportunity to introduce me to an ayurvedic humoral assessment of health problems. Diabetes, he stated, was a very imprecise allopathic disease category, and he expressed concern about a one-size-fits-all biomedical approach to treating diabetes, stating that in his experience this often led to iatrogenic (or treatment-induced) complications. The vaidya diagnosed diabetes patients according to ayurvedic nosology and the diagnostic category of *premeha,* which encompasses urinary flow disorders as well as diabetes. Ayurveda describes twenty types of premeha, some of which are curable and others are not. Each type is associated with a different type of humoral (*dosha*) imbalance. Treatment is tailored to both a patient's dosha imbalance and body type. Individuals who are obese (*sthula*) or lean (*krisha*) for reasons related to constitution, food habits, and lifestyle are treated differently, and the vaidya often asked them different types of questions while taking their histories.

One lesson the vaidya was intent on teaching me entailed an understanding of health as a dynamic state responsive to "action in the interaction" between body constitution, environment, and behavior. When he diagnosed patients, the vaidya took a detailed patient-centered history typically lasting more than an hour. During the consultation, he inquired not only about a patient's physical symptoms, which he read as signs of dosha imbalance, but also a patient's food habits and taste preferences, sleep patterns, sources of tension in their lives, and any and all things that might upset their digestion. The vaidya took pains to identify what I came to see as humoral-behavioral feedback loops. This appeared to be more challenging in the case of poor patients than obese middle-class patients, whom he typically had to wean off of a rich diet of sweet and oily foods as well as excessive medicines. An example is a feedback loop experienced by a poor farmer suffering from both premeha and depression-like symptoms. The farmer experienced "tension" linked to mounting debt he had incurred and to his inability to arrange his daughter's marriage. Tension resulted in poor sleep and increased consumption of beedi cigarettes and chewing tobacco as a means to do hard labor when he was tired. The vaidya pointed out to me how each of these factors were interrelated and how they all interfered with the patient's digestion, resulting in dosha imbalance, premaha, and psychological distress.[1] What he did not do was consider factors leading to rising debt among farmers or the proliferation of cheap tobacco products.

This brief vignette points out how noncommunicable diseases (NCDs) are recognized as biosocial disorders locally, and not just by public health researchers and social scientists. As social scientists of health and medicine, it is our charge to look beyond the biosocial disorders of individuals to larger trends. When viewing epidemics of NCDs such as diabetes, we must not only identify the groups at risk and study risky behavior, but also provide a systematic account of environments of risk and agents and policies that foster health disparity directly and indirectly.

Global rates of type 2 diabetes have risen so sharply in the last three decades that there is now debate on whether to classify the condition as an epidemic or a pandemic.[2] There are an estimated 382 million people worldwide who presently suffer from diabetes (90 percent from type 2 diabetes), with rates of diabetes rising faster in middle- and low-income countries (LMICs) than in the West. In 1980, the global prevalence rate of diabetes was 4.7 percent. By 2014, the global prevalence rate had climbed to 8.5 percent, with rates exceeding 14 percent among some indigenous groups and refugees subject to severe trauma and displacement.

It is well established that rising rates of type 2 diabetes are not merely a reflection of better knowledge and increased surveillance. This rapid rise in cases of type 2 diabetes is associated with both defective modernization and rising levels of insecurity among structurally vulnerable and displaced populations. In the literature, this spike in diabetes cases is most commonly linked to diabesity[3] and associated with globalization and industrialization, nutrition transition, the proliferation of obesogenic and other commerciogenic products (e.g., fast foods, tobacco, alcohol), and a sedentary lifestyle. Less often recognized, but equally important as risk factors, are chronic undernutrition and prolonged and pronounced periods of psychosocial stress, anxiety, and depression.[4] Type 2 diabetes is a preeminent stage four of epidemiological transition and it is contributing to the double burden of noncommunicable and communicable diseases in LMICs.[5]

Rethinking Diabetes shows very clearly how diabetes is rarely experienced as a stand-alone health problem. Aside from causing a wide spectrum of complications (e.g., heart disease, chronic ulcers, blindness), diabetes is comorbid with other NCDs ranging from hypertension and depression to polycystic ovary syndrome and dementia. Diabetes also compromises the immune system, rendering one far more vulnerable to infections such as *streptococcus pneumonia*, influenza virus, tuberculosis, and urinary tract infections. On the other hand, the likelihood that someone afflicted with HIV will experience diabetes is much greater than among the general population, as a result of insulin resistance associated with both the disease and its standard treatment.[6]

Rethinking Diabetes and other work by Emily Mendenhall argue that it is more productive to think about diabetes in terms of syndemics than of comorbidity or multimorbidity.[7] This line of critical biological investigation focuses on synergistic, not just concurrent, health problems and societal determinants of chronic ill health. In this book, Mendenhall expands her systematically documented and theoretically rigorous study of diabetes presented in *Syndemic Suffering* (2012) to reflect on other diabetes syndemics experienced by impoverished populations in different ecosocial and cultural contexts. Her most compelling cases involve women experiencing diabetes while trying to "make do" in adverse conditions. These women suffer high allostatic loads associated with unpredictability in their daily lives, competing demands for resources, gender role obligations, domestic conflicts, and violence in its many forms. For these women, diabetes is experienced and understood as a life (course) lesion[8] and the result of long-standing and pernicious biopsychosocial weathering. Thus, Mendenhall reminds us that a syndemic approach to diabetes would go beyond the monitoring of blood sugar levels to consider reasons for poor dietary and medicine adherence, sources of psychosocial stress leading to depression, patterns of tobacco and other drug use, and so on.

Rethinking Diabetes is timely and thought provoking. Diabetes is a massive global health challenge for which there is no magic bullet and for which no one-size-fits-all program is likely to be effective. As aptly noted by the vaidya introduced at the beginning of this preface, type 2 diabetes is not a single phenomenon. Mendenhall's book describes, through ethnographic vignettes in four contexts, how treatment programs will need to be tailored to different types of patients with different needs and access to different sets of material resources and levels of social support. In short, nations preparing to introduce new NCD programs will need to address diabetes syndemics as biosocial epiphenomena.

ACKNOWLEDGMENTS

Most books take years to come together and this one is no exception. I first began asking about the complicated, interlinking experiences of trauma, mental illness, and diabetes in 2007 in the Chicago kitchens of Mexican immigrants with diabetes. The stories, knowledge, and pastries consumed during those curious hours laid the groundwork for this study—and I am most indebted to those twenty-six people who introduced food for thought. Over the course of a decade, I have interviewed hundreds of people in four countries and am indebted to the hours they spent with me as well as to my research assistants. This book would be nothing if it were not for their stories.

The Chicago project would have been impossible without the patience and careful guidance of my mentor at Cook County Hospital, Elizabeth Jacobs. I am indebted to Veronica Delgado Hernandez and Sam Del Pozo, who provided critical institutional and social support, in addition to my administrative friends: Funeka, Audrean, Manju, Pawal, George, and Francisco. Also, I will never forget the kindness and flexibility the clinical staff offered me during my work in the General Medicine Clinic. The research was made possible by generous funding from the National Science Foundation and Northwestern University's Institute for Policy Research and The Graduate School. Deborah Winslow, Eliza Earle, Katie Clarke-Myers, Tracy Tohtz, Susan Higgins, and Dana Adam Fuller made grant application and management navigable. The Department of Anthropology at Northwestern University provided foundational training at the intersection of culture and biology; thank you especially to Rebecca Seligman, Thomas McDade, and Bill Leonard for your mentorship.

The Delhi project would have been impossible without the unwavering support and guidance of Dorairaj Prabhakaran at the Public Health Foundation of India (PHFI) and the Centre for Chronic Disease Control (CCDC). I was also grateful for the mentorship from Nikhil Tandon and partnerships with Roopa Shivashankar, Shweta Khandelwal, Kavita Singh, Preet Dhillon, and others during my time in Delhi. The work would not have been possible without the research team for the CARRS study and Roopa's guidance. Our research assistants, Sneha Kamal Sharma and Allam Ashraf, made this research a success by conducting interviews with scientific rigor, patient persistence, and compassion. Others who made this research possible include PHFI and CCDC staff, especially Suma and Kamala. I was supported during this time as a Fogarty International Clinical Research Scholar with the National Institutes of Health. I am grateful for the support of the Vanderbilt University Institute for Global Health for managing this fellowship, including Sten Vermund, Doug Heimburger, Catherine Lem Carothers, Annie Smart, and Sarah Schlachter. Special thanks to Mohammed K. Ali and K.M. Venkat Narayan for selecting me to be Emory University's NIH Fogarty Scholar and for allowing me the intellectual freedom to do something new. Finally, a special thank you to Lesley Jo Weaver, whose advice on working as an anthropologist on diabetes in Delhi was critical to my success; I continue to value our friendship and collaborative work.

The Soweto project was successful due to Shane Norris's courage and flexibility to welcome an ethnographic perspective into the Development Pathways for Health Research Unit (DPHRU) at the University of the Witwatersrand. It was a privilege to work with Shane and others who continue the work on the cohort study initially known as Mandela's Children. I was also grateful for the guidance from other postdoctoral fellows, including

Alison Feeley, and staff, including Prisha, Jorris, Nelson, Rhulani, Thabile, Lisa, and Mat. Mama Hunadi Shawa and Meikie Hlalele assisted with eight interviews conducted in Soweto with individuals who preferred their native language to English. Mama Hunadi also recruited women to speak with us, managed logistics, and engaged with me in lengthy discussions about women's stories. The research and opportunity to work with DPHRU would have been impossible without the financial support of South Africa's Medical Research Council and the support and flexibility of the research team. Finally, our time in South Africa was made especially sweet by living with the Mallen family and running with Team Kudu.

The Nairobi project was successful on account of the seamless support from David Ndetei and Victoria Mutiso at the Africa Mental Health Foundation (AMHF). I am indebted to Abednego Musau, who played a fundamental role in getting the research off the ground. Edna Bosire, Gitonga Isaiah, and Gregory Barnabas Omondi are three researchers who went above and beyond the expectations of this project. They are intelligent, committed, and fun to be around—it is a privilege to watch their careers take off since our first time working together. It was their curiosity and commitment to the project that enabled us to move quickly from data to publication and to engage deeply. The research was made possible by my generous start-up research funds from the School of Foreign Service at Georgetown University—I am especially appreciative of the institutional support from Jennifer Long, Obdulio Moronta, and Nicholas Starvaggi. Notably, my family is indebted to Kate and Oliver Sabot for opening their home and filling our bellies with a great deal of laughter, adventure, and good food. A special thanks to Jane for caring for our little Fiona during our months in Nairobi.

Amidst the multisited research was a strong network of scholars who have influenced the ideas in this book. There will never be enough thanks for Peter J. Brown, who first introduced me to medical anthropology and continues to be a treasured mentor. My cadre of colleagues and friends whom I met over a decade ago at Emory University continue to inspire and shape my research and intellectual growth, including Sarah S. Willen, Erin Finley Garcia, Kenneth Maes, Jed Stevenson, Svea Closser, Brandon Kohrt, Ryan Brown, Sarah Raskin, Lesley Jo Weaver, and Jennifer Kuzara. Other medical anthropologists who have been especially kind to think through these ideas with me include Sara Lewis and Lauren Carruth.

My new academic home, Georgetown University, welcomed me with open arms and has become a bastion of intellectual growth and political engagement. I am grateful for my wonderful colleagues in the Science, Technology, and International Affairs program, including Mark Giordano, Joanna Lewis, Kathy Olesko, Sarah Stewart Johnson, and Rajesh Veerarahgavan. I have been privileged to engage and learn from my colleagues in African Studies, and especially Lahra Smith, a collaborator and friend. Moreover, the Department of Anthropology has provided a warm welcome and continual friendship. The global health community that spans the campus has also been an important cornerstone—special thanks to John Monahan for engaging repeatedly to discuss global health policy. Finally, this project would have been inconceivable without the loving support for my kids by the wonderful staff at Hoya Kids Learning Center. I want especially to thank Jane, Susan, Molly, Sarah, Liz, Todd, Yanka, Mary Kate, Aleria, Tanya, Vikki, Jenn, Sharon, NuNu, Chris, Katie, and Hannah.

A group of incredibly insightful scholars pushed this book from a collection of four discrete ethnographic case studies into an integrated story. Thank you Lenore Manderson and Janet McGrath for your critical push for a major rewrite and extensive comments. Thank you to Abraham Newman and the Mortara Center for International Studies at Georgetown for financing a book workshop and to Janet McGrath, Heide Castañeda, Daniel J. Smith, Lauren Carruth, Lahra Smith, Sara Lewis, Rajesh Veeraraghavan, Brandon Kohrt, and Jennifer Huang Bouey for engaging in a full day of constructive and clarifying critique. Also, thank you to Jessica Yen, H. Stowe McMurry, and Shelby Rowler for jumping in to help me at critical moments.

There will never be enough thanks for my family. My parents, Walter and Barbara, set a high bar for what incredibly supportive parenting can be. Kate and Zach are unfailing in their support—and especially in their encouragement to turn it off and jump in Lake Okoboji. My Aunt Abby read numerous versions of what is in these pages. Many others challenged me to think about the questions in this book. Most importantly, they encouraged me to flip off my computer to enjoy a sweaty hike, a swim in refreshing waters, a good book, and stimulating conversation.

Adam is the type of person who makes me laugh so much my stomach hurts. Belly laughs, parenting, travelling, researching, writing, hiking, thinking, kayaking, drinking wine, taking a run, or taking a break—everything is better with you. I am so lucky to share these things, as well as our continuous dialogue and work together around the world, which is the essence of the pages in this book. Along the way, welcoming our little people, Fiona and Zoë, has been the source of incredible love and resounding joy. May they see in their lifetimes a safer, more just world for women, our planet, and humankind, everywhere.

In what follows, all errors are mine alone.

RETHINKING DIABETES

INTRODUCTION

Esther

Esther awoke with the sun, paid the bus fare, and arrived early as the gate opened at the district hospital. Patients milled around the specialty clinic waiting room—a porch nestled within tall beams and a tin roof. Esther sat outside along the dusty path that wove through the hospital compound. Some, like Esther, were there seeking care for their diabetes. Some had tuberculosis. Others had cancer. They sat together on the closely spaced benches as cool breeze chilled the air. She wrapped her blanket around her tightly and looked at the other patients.

Esther edged away from her neighbor, who had started coughing. She worried he had tuberculosis—something she should not catch, as she was taking antiretrovirals (ARVs) for HIV, and now diabetes symptoms were making her feel sick. In the past year, Esther suffered from bouts of malaria and typhoid as well. These acute infections complicated her severe and at time disabling depression, which washed over her during the most difficult times.

Much later in the day, Esther spent hours sharing her story in a quiet open-air tent outside the clinic. The tent was situated on the edge of the medical compound on a grassy knoll. From her perch, the specialty clinic was in sight, and by darting her eyes she saw the stand-alone building for patients who were HIV positive. She had received antiretroviral therapy (ART) there during past visits.

Esther was born in 1962 in rural western Kenya to a Kikuyu family of humble means. She lived with her mother, father, and twelve siblings in a small traditional home. When her father died of alcoholism when she was in primary school, her situation changed dramatically and forced her family off their land. Esther explained that her father died "before he got a share of his ancestral land." This drove her family into absolute poverty and homelessness. Her mother moved the family to a coffee plantation and tea farm, what she describes as the "white settler's lands," to look for work; there, they "were given tents or temporary houses for workers." Few of Esther's siblings showed interest in school, and she was the only one to complete five years of free primary education. She spoke longingly of one teacher who encouraged her to complete her schooling. Like her other siblings, however, Esther was needed to earn money to support her family, and eventually she joined her siblings in the fields. She recollected that her mother "did not want to lose labor in the farms."

Esther left the rural area for Nairobi in her twenties. Her mother remains in a rural area with six of Esther's living siblings; six others died years ago from AIDS. Many were infected in the 1980s and 1990s, years before ART became widely available for treatment of those with HIV. Such treatment was especially difficult for low-income families like Esther's. She explained, "One of my sisters got HIV when she was in standard seven [one year before completing primary school]. She decided to get married, but unfortunately she got infected with HIV. She later died." Esther stated that it was by caring for her sick siblings that she became HIV positive. She went on: "You see, in those days there were no ARVs and people did not have knowledge about how to prevent HIV transmission. After my sisters died, I got tested and I was diagnosed with HIV." Esther took her time with this memory, slowly revisiting the historical trauma and personal devastation inflicted by the AIDS epidemic on her family.

Esther fell into a deep depression after she was diagnosed with HIV. She noted that she felt hatred toward herself before she learned to accept her status. Esther entered a program to help others living with and grieving HIV and AIDS.[1] She became a community health worker through a European nongovernmental organization (NGO). In this work, Esther would "help those people infected by HIV and create awareness." She became one of the many HIV-positive volunteers who give their time and energy for little (and, in some cases, no) pay. Esther was paid 2,000 Kenyan shillings per month ($20). She used this money to "buy food for the sick and poor people, because even with the introduction of ARVs, some patients were so poor and bedridden that they could not have food to eat before they took their medications. So, I bought them food."

During this time Esther married and had four children. After fifteen years, however, Esther's marriage dissolved abruptly, the result of an infidelity that left indelible marks in her life. Her husband "took advantage of" her younger sister, and they had a child. This hurt her deeply and, as tradition requires, Esther reported it to her in-laws' family. The family decided that they would take in Esther's younger sister as a co-wife because Esther's husband had enough money to support them both. Esther was devastated by both the infidelity and the violence against her sister. She said, "I could not accept this and I decided to leave with my four children and start my own life." She left her sister with her husband.

This is when Esther first moved to Kibera, the largest slum in the African continent. She "worked there as a bar attendant for eight years" and was able to "educate my children up to standard eight," which was the completion of primary school. She regretted that her children could not continue to secondary school because she had too little money to pay for their fees. Eventually, Esther met a man with whom she moved in and had three more children. At 52, she was determined for these three children to complete their secondary schooling.

Esther moved from Kibera to another low-income Nairobi neighborhood when she remarried. However, personal security in her new neighborhood proved to be a constant struggle. She said that "security is not so good" mostly because of "theft issues," because "boys are criminal and they steal from people." There were also serious issues related to gun violence that fostered chronic stress, as shown by her statement that "about seven of the boys were killed last year. They had guns that they used to terrorize people."

As many women do, Esther felt these social experiences deeply within her body, explaining: "All these things were so stressful that I developed wounds in my stomach." Like before, when she had struggled with the loss of her siblings, Esther found a counselor to speak with: "It took me about two years before I accepted my situation. I think I realized that in every situation, I had to accept my background and even my destiny. I did not choose to be born by poor parents. I was born there by accident. I had to accept all these things in my life."

Esther tested positive for HIV in 2002. At that time, however, she was healthy. After two years, she began taking Septrin, a broad-range antibiotic often used for diarrhea and urinary tract infections. Six years later, her CD4 count fell low enough that she began ART. She was also dealing with a noxious herpes outbreak and sought treatment. By 2008, ART was largely available in Kenya, and she was treated free of charge. The free clinic provided a comprehensive exam, including a blood test. During this appointment Esther discovered that she had diabetes, too. She went on to explain: "They only gave HIV services and treatment for free. Other diseases such as diabetes are paid for [by the patient]. This is making my life difficult because I can't afford these services." Money clearly matters in how she strategically cares for her multiple conditions: "I have used diabetic medications for about two years. Due to affordability issue, I am forced to skip diabetic medications."

Esther explained that diabetes escalated her HIV infection because it compromised her immunity. She explained: "My CD4 went down and the doctor advised me to use ARVs because he told me that diabetes may affect my eyesight or other things." In many ways, Esther preferred HIV over diabetes: "The advantage with HIV is that the ARVs are available. But for diabetes, it is hard to get medications when one has no money to buy the drugs."

It is not, however, about only drugs. Esther explained that buying new foods was stressful and also affected her pocketbook: "Before, I used to buy food that would take us the whole month. But with diabetes, it needs a special diet, something that has strained my budget. It is also hard for poor people like us. I wish diabetes could be affecting the rich because they can afford special meals." She went on: "I sometimes skip diabetes medications due to lack of money. I also do farming and I get plenty vegetables but sometimes I have no money to buy brown flour and other foods. I also don't know much about fruits, I don't know which fruits are good and which ones are bad. I usually feel afraid when I am eating." She said that she felt "alone" with diabetes. "Today at the clinic," she explained, "I have been told to start using insulin. The doctor has told me to keep the medicines in the fridge. But you see, I even have no electricity. I also have no fridge."

Global Diabetes

In the past several decades, diabetes has traveled across the globe.[2] Many have argued that the proliferation of diabetes in unexpected communities like Esther's punctuates the rapid nutrition transition fostered by the unbridled corporate expansion of the food industry. This story illustrates what was initially described by Syndey Mintz (1985) as a marriage of sugar and capitalism, that is, a relationship defined by exploitative labor in the sugar industry that is further driven by the poor's heavy consumption of sugar and the wealthy's extraordinary financial benefit from it.[3] Many anthropologists and epidemiologists use this narrative to explain how neoliberal capitalism has driven the nutrition transition across the globe and from wealthy to poorer communities.[4] Yet, defining global diabetes simply as a product of modernization overlooks the complex cultural, social, and biological dimensions that drive and situate the epidemic differently across contexts. As Emily Yates-Doerr (2015, 52) describes in relation to her scholarship on obesity and diabetes in Guatemala, "rather than understand modernity as a looming urban future (contrasted with a traditional, rural past), the modernity of relevance . . . [is] woven into various places and various times, moving in and out of relevance in different situated ways." This book investigates the complex, divergent ways in which global and local factors transform how diabetes becomes embodied and experienced from place to place.

Historically, 90 percent of individuals living with diabetes have been classified with type 2, or adult-onset, diabetes.[5] This type usually develops later in life, which flashes a light on the potential ecological, social, and biological factors that produce diabetes. Many have associated this type of diabetes with widening waistlines, using the idiom "diabesity" to emphasize how commonly obesity and diabetes travel together.[6] Although expanding waistlines are one of the most powerful predictors of diabetes, people with diabetes are increasingly thinner and younger than in previous decades, with complex co-occurring conditions including depression, hypertension, and, more recently, infections like HIV and tuberculosis. This is one reason some scholars contend that there is more biological variation in diabetes than was previously conceived.[7] This suggests not only that the condition differs metabolically across the globe but also that factors apart from obesity are driving the condition and creating new challenges for people with diabetes.[8] This is especially true for those communities who face the most arduous political and social inequalities, as those who are low income are increasingly the most afflicted.[9] Yet, because half of the cases go undiagnosed in such contexts, many seek medical care only when they become very sick.[10]

I argue that neoliberal capitalism becomes a companion to the intrinsic links between hunger and crisis, structural violence and fear, and cumulative trauma and psychiatric distress that are embodied in diabetes. In some sense, the diabetes crisis has been provoked by governments prioritizing profits over people. This can be traced to the failure of national governments to regulate what foods are available and at what price. The global flows of food and the replacement of organic, fresh, and healthy foods with quick, fried, and processed foods that fill people's bellies with few nutrients are powerful conduits of diabetes.[11] Yet, diabetes is also closely aligned to historical legacies of systemic oppression, from enslavement to displacement and segregation, as communities who have long been oppressed due to ethnicity, race, and class are the most affected by diabetes.[12] Such processes frame the embodied stress associated with meeting the demands of quickening lifestyles and increasing food prices and the need to keep one's family safe, fed, loved, and warm. A global story of modernization disregards the structural dimensions that drive the underlying psychophysiological processes linking hunger, crisis, oppression, and unbridled stress to diabetes. The narratives in this book unveil how deeply embedded such factors are in how diabetes is experienced and (re)produced among poor communities around the world.

The story of Native Americans and diabetes exemplifies how centuries of systematic oppression can produce unprecedented levels of diabetes.[13]

Whereas one in three children born in the United States is estimated to develop diabetes at some point in life, among many Native American communities that probability is higher than one in two.[14] For instance, consider the case of the Pima, an indigenous community in the United States and Mexico partitioned by the U.S.-Mexico border nearly a century ago. Some reside on reservations in the United States, and others reside just across the border in Mexico. Those residing in Arizona were forcibly resettled onto a reservation in order to construct a hydraulic dam and reservoir in 1924, whereas most Pima in Mexico continued farming and raising livestock. Consequently, the Pima in Arizona have long relied on ration cards and food subsidies for mostly calorie-dense, low-quality, highly processed foods. The vastly different histories, social conditions, diets, and lifestyles among the Pima have shaped disparities in their experiences of diabetes as well. The Pima living in the United States have experienced significantly more diabetes and obesity in the past several decades[15] compared to those in Mexico (although obesity and diabetes are pervasive in Mexico, too).[16] This discrepancy illustrates the link between poor diet, obesity, and diabetes. However, the trauma of forced relocation and fragmented social worlds cannot be removed from this story, because real biological and pathological pathways of trauma and chronic stress, from epigenetics to psychophysiology, lead to diabetes.[17]

Although social and political histories differ dramatically, Esther's story reflects similar forms of colonialism and embodied trauma. In the shadow of British colonialism, Esther's displacement from her home and school, the loss of her father, and the experience of child labor curbed her opportunities to thrive from the beginning. These obstacles not only made financial insecurity chronic but also provoked an internalization of the persistent emotional pain that trailed her childhood. This early suffering was soon met by the AIDS epidemic, which torched her family as Esther nursed her siblings to their deaths and was eventually infected. These experiences occurred amid her husband's infidelities and eventual demise from AIDS. Esther carried this emotional pain with her for many years and experienced deep anxiety and depression. These were compounded by constant financial insecurity, such as the lack of a functioning fridge to keep insulin fresh. The consumption of foods and pharmaceuticals for her multiple conditions also created challenges for diabetes self-care. These complex dynamics were driven by global health politics that shape local health systems, determining which drugs she could and could not access, as well as by the trade-offs she made between taking care of her loved ones and taking care of her body when she felt bad.

Despite these extraordinary setbacks, Esther was not defeated and in fact demonstrated admirable strength. Her courage to care for her loved ones during the height of the impact of the AIDS epidemic on her family revealed not only deep love but also concern for those around her. Unlike many in similar situations, Esther sought counseling after this traumatic life period, which brought relief to the distress in her body. Similarly, when confronted with her husband's infidelity and violence, she left him, taking her children with her (though not without some regret). She showed courage when confronted with tough choices. As a community health worker, moreover, Esther gained emancipatory knowledge about life-saving medication that prolonged her life by decades. Importantly, this knowledge gives new significance to the trade-offs Esther frequently made between food and diabetes care: Her decision to take diabetes medications only when she felt bad reveals calculated choices weighing the risk to her body against the risk of not feeding her family (as opposed to a simpler understanding of biomedical "risk"). Making sense of how people navigate risk and compliance amid crippling financial insecurity challenges moral authorities that use compliance to determine who is "good" or "bad" at caring for diabetes.[18]

Life stories like Esther's make evident the need to revise prevailing narratives about global diabetes. In doing so, we must take seriously how the social pathways revealed in Esther's story become transduced into the biological risk that so commonly undergirds diabetes. For instance, trauma from childhood (such as physical or sexual violence) that persists years later in daily life cannot be dissociated from the chronic stress and inflammation within the body that are dually linked to diabetes.[19] Immigrating away from one's loved ones cannot be dissociated from some people's deep depression, sadness, or grief.[20] Changes in family structure that leave some women alone or responsible for caregiving for multiple dependents—from grandchildren to spouses—cannot be dissociated from the financial and social strains that lead to persistent anxiety, neglected diets, skipped medications, or difficulties making it to the clinic.[21] Taking ART and living with HIV has been associated with increased risk for diabetes.[22] These challenges are furthered by feeling unsafe within one's home or neighborhood, which produces a chronic hypervigilance.[23] Stress hormones also rage beneath untreated emotional pain that is expressed in local idioms of distress, somatic pain, and psychiatric distress.[24] The crippling financial insecurity reflected in the lack of a functioning fridge to keep foods fresh and insulin cold further confounds people's experiences of diabetes.[25]

Understanding how these complex social, political, psychological, and biological pathways weave together demands a synergistic interpretation. I argue that among socially and economically vulnerable communities like Esther's, diabetes always exists syndemically. First conceptualized by the critical medical anthropologist Merrill Singer (1994, 1996, 2003, 2006, 2009), a syndemic describes how social and health conditions travel together through a population, interact in meaningful ways via social, biological, or psychological pathways, and are driven by social and political forces. I return to syndemic diabetes, and particularly a theory of syndemic suffering, in chapter 1. I argue that syndemic theory provides an interdisciplinary voice for thinking about how diabetes materializes across populations while taking seriously the complex ways in which metabolic experiences sit in the lives of individuals and communities.

The Project

Anthropological scholarship on diabetes and social suffering has focused on the complicated interactions of political marginalization, racism, classism, and sexism at work, at home, and in the clinic.[26] Jo Scheder (1988) was one of the first anthropologists to argue that social suffering was inherently embedded in diabetes in her research among Mexican farmworkers in the United States. Scheder illustrated how the compounded effect of life's challenges was a greater contributor to glucose intolerance than obesity or perceived stress. Melanie Rock (2003) leveraged the weight of social suffering on diabetes while discussing why three in five of Canada's First Nation people have diabetes compared to much lower rates in the general population; she attributed disparity to social distress and duress and underscored lived experiences as paramount in diabetes. Others, such as Carolyn Smith-Morris (2008) and Dennis Wiedman (2012), have illuminated how histories of political marginalization, physical confinement to reservation lands, and government-subsidized food and medical programs have contributed to a remarkably high prevalence of gestational and type 2 diabetes among Native Americans. Mariana Ferreira and Gretchen Lang (2006) argue further that among indigenous people throughout the world—who are disproportionately afflicted by the disease—diabetes reflects the violence and oppression of colonialism, displacement, and cultural expansionism. Recent monographs by Emily Yates-Doerr (2015), Megan Carney (2015), and Harris Solomon (2016) have claimed that neoliberal economic realities produce the complicated interactions of food, substances, and ideas that become revealed in the metabolic heterogeneities, including diabetes, that cannot be dislocated from global change but produce uniquely local realities. In these ways, which largely attend to biological or clinical aspects, as opposed to biomedical frameworks, anthropological perspectives on diabetes examine how the disease is inherently social and rooted in historical landscapes of oppression and subjugation from colonialism, segregation, and neoliberalism. These studies reveal trends in diabetes that extend across the globe.

This scholarship inspired my previous multimethod, multiyear study of trauma and diabetes among Mexican immigrant women seeking care at a large public hospital clinic in Chicago, a large, diverse, and segregated city in the United States.[27] In Chicago, the chronicities of poverty, immigration stress, abuse, and depression among Mexican immigrant women with diabetes were so pervasive that I argued that these factors clustered together to create syndemic suffering. I also found that people tended to use their diabetes to communicate complexities of social trauma, poverty, and mental illness that were transduced into their metabolic experiences. In fact, I argued that diabetes became an idiom of distress—functioning as a "narrative wedge" for talking about emotional distress.[28] These narratives exemplified how diabetes was a function of poverty and structural violence and how social traumas and psychological suffering were deeply embedded not only in insulin resistance as a biological marker of diabetes but also in diabetes as a social and cultural experience.

The global scope of the current project was inspired by an invitation to spend a year in Delhi, India. After thinking seriously about how social suffering produces diabetes in Chicago, I was intrigued to learn more about how diabetes was differently experienced and embodied among people of different economic backgrounds in Delhi—the capital city of what was at the time the nation with the second largest population living with diabetes in the world.[29] In Delhi I investigated how social, political, economic, and cultural factors shape diabetes experiences across socioeconomic groups by interviewing people residing in wealthy, middle-class, and low-income neighborhoods. I organized the study to investigate how income might transform how people experience changing dynamics of food, family, belief, and emotion and how these may reflect metabolic heterogeneities as well as care-seeking for diabetes. For instance, the foods people eat in Delhi often are linked to income, as are the modes of transportation people use, from cars to rickshaws, and the spaces people inhabit within the city, from luxury condos to cramped one-bedroom apartments.[30] Although I focus mostly on the experiences of low-income women living with diabetes and social and economic stress, I also consider how poverty and wealth influence how people think about, interact with, and seek care for diabetes in Delhi.

After a year in Delhi, I wanted to return to sub-Saharan Africa to better understand the swiftly escalating numbers of people living with diabetes there. I had spent time in southern Africa a decade earlier, and at the time diabetes was almost never mentioned in my research at an HIV clinic. Yet increasing epidemiological evidence was now pointing to an escalation of diabetes in South Africa, a middle-income country, which reflected a legacy of deep-seated racial segregation and health inequities not unlike those found in the United States. Moreover, diabetes was increasingly observed among low-income urban communities in South Africa[31] that were dually afflicted by HIV and AIDS. My interest in where, how, and among whom diabetes was emerging in such contexts was informed in part by Didier Fassin's (2009) scholarship, which argues that the deeply rooted structures of inequality of apartheid contributed significantly to the uneven distribution of HIV among the population. In the country most affected by HIV and AIDS in the world, carrying 17 percent of the global burden, what did the emergence of diabetes mean among the communities most afflicted by HIV? I was also curious to see how people navigated diabetes in the face of HIV. How did people conceive of a chronic illness that was relatively new? How might HIV and diabetes afflict similar communities, families, and individuals? How might these two chronic illnesses interact?[32]

The final stop on my journey was at a public hospital clinic in Nairobi, Kenya, a context where still very little was known about who was affected by diabetes or how it was perceived or experienced. One study suggested that diabetes was salient in urban slums, and many assumed this to be the case. Working at a public hospital clinic near Kibera (the largest informal settlement, or slum, in Nairobi), I crafted questions that sought to get at the heart of how people *perceived* and *experienced* the binaries and intersections of HIV and diabetes that are exemplified in narratives like Esther's. By casting a wider net of potential interlocutors, I was able to interrogate how the HIV-diabetes convergence affects one's social and medical experiences. In this study—more than any other—the financing of diabetes care (or the lack thereof) played a central role in how people perceived diabetes and juxtaposed it to HIV. Because Kenya relies substantially on donor assistance to strengthen its health system, this finding introduced an interesting twist. It also shed a light on how complicated international donor policies can become when implemented into a public hospital context: Esther and others explicitly demonstrated how such policies framed their own perception and experience of diabetes. Thus, these narratives brought new dimensions of health system impacts to the surface, moving beyond the clinic and into the broader sphere of global health and development priorities.

Methods

This book is fundamentally a cross-cultural analysis of diabetes experiences. Thus, I have tried to be self-reflective enough to prevent the potential mishap of what Arjun Appadurai (1986, 361) has called the "arbitrary hegemony" of regions in anthropological theory building. In this sense, I take seriously the ethnographic descriptions that I have collected and try to build as robust a comparative perspective as possible while recognizing that my samples are small and findings are locally contingent. In doing so, I emphasize that place matters for a careful study of diabetes and social suffering. This has resulted in a comparative analysis of what defines suffering in everyday lives, how such experiences become syndemic, and how the convergence of ideas, lived lives, and epidemiological realities move within and beyond the forums of anthropological thought.

I use narrative as the primary path for discussing diabetes and experience across cultures. Throughout the book, I employ the terms "story," "narrative," and "life history narrative" interchangeably. I use the story as a central orienting tool because stories have long held a central place in anthropology—from studies of ritual to analyses of belief, space, illness, and experience.[33] In particular, stories have been fundamental to the study of chronic illness, from Gay Becker's (1997) study of disrupted lives to Sue Estroff's (1993) reflections on chronicity and Cheryl Mattingly's (1998) analysis of clinical plots.[34] Situating my use of narratives is imperative because stories were the crux of my research but not the exclusive data collected or prioritized. I collected data through multiple and mixed methods, including surveys, psychiatric inventories, anthropometrics, and biological data.[35] The reflective memory work that is generated through storytelling provided an opportunity to interpret what Rebecca Seligman (2010, 298) has called the "embodied self." These narratives integrate personal experience with psychological and biological responses to reveal how culture, society, and biology become embodied in a complicated life story. Hence, the use of mixed methods has enabled me to juxtapose the subjectivities of narrative with psychological and physical symptoms of distress, generating a theory of syndemic suffering that is subjectively defined, contextually rooted, and communicated through the mind and body.

I also draw heavily on Eleanor Ochs and Lisa Capps's (2001, 2) interpretation of the living narrative, which they describe as what happens when people come together to "build accounts of life events." This differs significantly from a polished story with a beginning, a middle, and an end built into a chronological design. Instead, these stories arise through a framing of life by way of "conversational narrative [that] will include questions, clarifications, challenges and speculations" (2001, 19). The narratives collected for this book were not rehearsed, and most likely many of the stories had not been shared often, especially those about the more intimate and sometimes traumatic periods of people's lives. However, this is not a book about the intricacies of how a story is told. Instead, I use individual stories to draw out what key cultural and personal references people prioritize when remembering a life, and what forms of suffering and resilience are used to make meaning out of a life remembered.

The Data

I was first intrigued by what drives diabetes when I asked Mexican immigrant women about their diabetes experiences in Chicago. When speaking about their diabetes, most women emphasized other forms of social and psychological suffering. I found this fascinating because it flipped the biomedical model for diabetes on its head. I began to understand how the clinical world in which I had been working oversold the individual, behavioral interventions of diet and exercise. However, I did not yet understand the extent to which they were misguided. My interlocutors eloquently conveyed how such prescriptions were nearly impossible to comply with due to cost, fear, stress, and the challenge of filling their cupboards with the "right" foods. Of all the stressors in their life, diabetes was situated very low on their list of life's challenges. I was increasingly convinced that the narrow treatments for their condition were missing the point and causing them to become sicker.

In Chicago, I worked for five years on a study of culture, diabetes, and health care at the largest public hospital clinic in the city. I first conducted a small ethnographic study about diabetes beliefs and experiences in the home of twenty-six Mexican immigrants who routinely sought care at the clinic. I also participated in a larger survey of more than four hundred people living with diabetes and seeking care from the public hospital. Then, I developed an in-depth life history narrative interview combined with multiple surveys and biomarkers in order to better understand the lived experiences of trauma and diabetes among the Mexican immigrant women from the clinic. I conducted 121 four- to six-hour interviews in order to capture their lived experiences and to collect enough biological and psychiatric markers of distress to speak across disciplines. These stories were at the heart of my book *Syndemic Suffering,* and some of those ideas are incorporated into chapter 2.

The study methodology was similar in India, South Africa, and Kenya. I spent less time in these contexts, however, but worked closely with others and depended on my colleagues for linguistic, cultural, and political expertise. In Delhi, my team conducted sixty life history interviews with people with diabetes residing in three neighborhoods differing in wealth. These interlocutors were invited to participate because they were enrolled in the CARRS Cohort Study,[36] which involved more than 5,000 households. In Johannesburg, my team conducted twenty-seven interviews among women residing in Soweto, a low-income neighborhood where the Birth to Twenty Plus Cohort had followed more than 1,000 families for more than two decades.[37] These interlocutors were recruited from that study, where they figured as caregivers of the children enrolled in the study. Finally, in Nairobi, my team conducted one hundred interviews with patients seeking care at a public hospital clinic near Kibera, including Esther's interview.[38]

In this book, I primarily focus on the narratives collected during the small ethnographic studies conducted in parallel with other larger projects.[39] Table 1 shows the similarities in age and income across study sites as well as the differences in volume, ethnicity, and gender. For instance, in Chicago and Nairobi I collected all levels of data presented in this book; in Soweto and Delhi, by contrast, some biological, survey, and anthropometric data were drawn from parent cohort studies. Table 2 outlines parallels between studies as well as divergent modes through which I assessed life history narratives and survey, psychiatric, anthropometric, and biological data (which are described in detail in each chapter).

These independent studies reflect one another in many ways. First, most of my interlocutors were women living with diabetes. I interviewed 121 women in Chicago, 29 in Delhi, 27 in Soweto, and 50 in Nairobi (n = 227). One-fourth of the life stories I collected were with men, with 30 interviewed in Delhi and 50 in Nairobi (n = 80). In Delhi I interviewed people across the socioeconomic strata; of these only 20 were low income, and of these only 11 were women. In Nairobi half of the participants were recruited from a primary care clinic and were the only people in the whole study without a diabetes diagnosis (although most were insulin resistant). Second, nearly all of my interlocutors resided in low-income neighborhoods. Most Mexican immigrant women in Chicago resided in hyper-segregated impoverished neighborhoods. Interlocutors in Delhi

TABLE 1. Sociodemographics

	Location	Age	Income	Ethnicity	Language	Enrolled	Diabetes diagnosed	Women
United States	Chicago	40–65	Low	Mexican	Spanish, English	121	121	121
India	Delhi	35–70	Mixed	Mixed	Hindi	60	60	30
South Africa	Soweto	40–65	Low	Mixed	Zulu, Sesotho, English	27	27	27
Kenya	Nairobi	35–70	Low	Mixed	Kiswahili	100	50	50

TABLE 2. Mixed Methods Across Contexts

	United States	India	South Africa	Kenya
Life history narratives	✓	✓	✓	✓
Sociodemographics	✓	✓	✓	✓
Stress scales	✓			
Depression inventory	✓	✓		✓
Anxiety inventory				✓
PTSD inventory	✓			
General psychiatric inventory			✓	
Disease checklist			✓	✓
Hemoglobin A1c	✓	✓	✓	✓
Blood pressure	✓	✓	✓	✓
Body mass index	✓	✓	✓	✓
Independent study	✓			✓
Cohort parent study		✓	✓	

were divided by neighborhoods, with one group living in an affluent area, one in a middle-class neighborhood, and another identified as primarily residing in government housing. Most individuals featured in this book were relocated from slums to reside in government housing, but I do speak across socioeconomic groups. Those interviewed in Soweto and Kibera (within Johannesburg and Nairobi, respectively) resided in low-income neighborhoods known locally as townships or slums. Third, nearly everyone in this study was older than 35 years of age and younger than 70 years. Most participants were between the ages of 40 and 65, which was orchestrated in the study design because this is the age range in which diabetes and co-occurring depression tend to flourish. Finally, in each site I approached the study in a similar way, by placing life history narratives at the center and unpacking the complexities behind those stories with data on stress, psychology, and biology. The measures may vary slightly as a result of collaborator research priorities, available measures, and laboratory capabilities, but the data provide a platform to compare the different entanglements within people's lives.

When I compare study sites, I focus my discussion on the low-income women with diabetes who participated in each project. Throughout the book, I refer to those individuals who struggled each day to pay their rent, feed their families, and clothe their children as "low-income" and "the poor"; I use these terms to emphasize the relative economic insecurity of their situation. Their suffering, however, differs across locales, and the diversity found within these four sites provides insight into how local factors shape diabetes.

The comparative data also open up opportunities to think about how intersectionalities[40] of gender, class, social trauma, negative emotion, and chronicity become embodied in health and illness. Marcia Inhorn (2006, 361) emphasizes the importance of thinking about intersectionality in women's health, underscoring the "interlocking nature of various forms of oppression." The anthropologist Leith Mullings (2005, 80) has pioneered such work, arguing that "interlocking, interactive, and relational categories" must seek to understand how the axes of stratification intersect at certain historical moments and across various "health disparities, structural vulnerability, and [sources of] resilience." Recognizing such oppression as violence underscores how stratifications based on gender, race, ethnicity, class, and/or sexuality become normalized, symbolic, or, to use a term from Veena Das (2006, 2008, 2015), "ordinary." Thus, these normalized forms of oppression as well as resilience find an expression in the reflective memory work conveyed throughout this book.

The Chapters

Chapter 1 begins with the story of María, a Mexican immigrant in Chicago who faces complex social demands while confronting new frontiers of independence and chronic illness. The story is intended to open a discussion on social suffering, power, and the variations of "global" and "local" that transform everyday lives and become realized in different experiences of diabetes. In doing so, I address multiple layers of scholarship and bring together anthropological, public health, medical, and biological perspectives. Most of this research—like María's story—comes from wealthy nations; therefore, I comment on how diabetes and its partners in such contexts differ from their counterparts in lower-income countries. Weaving between multiple layers of knowledge and understanding of diabetes, this chapter makes the important point that structural violence, social experiences, and interpersonal relationships play a fundamental role in how diabetes is experienced and expressed across cultures, especially among the poor.

Chapter 2 centers around Beatriz, a Mexican immigrant woman with diabetes. This narrative reveals what I call the VIDDA syndemic, which compounds the impacts of structural violence, immigration, depression, diabetes, and abuse over the life course to shape women's suffering. For instance, multiple traumatic experiences of immigration across the US-Mexico border frame many women's stories, causing worry and persistent, untreated distress. Beatriz and others shared how other social traumas, including violence within the domestic and public spheres, continue to torment their minds and build up in their bodies. This chapter uses women's narratives to systematically demonstrate how these social and psychological factors define their chronic illness and how depression and diabetes are intimately connected in their everyday negotiations of foods, pharmaceuticals, and self-care. Beatriz's narrative emphasizes further how fundamentally linked financial security and health security become in everyday life.

Chapter 3 introduces Meena, a Hindu woman residing in a government housing settlement in north Delhi. She faces the challenges of diabetes, personal distress, and social pressures linked with social mobility and financial insecurity. For instance, the intergenerational stress associated with joint-family living arrangements fuels memories of suffering at the hands of her mother-in-law, but at the same time it allows Meena to develop survival strategies through the support of her daughter-in-law. While articulating swift-changing cultural norms, this chapter also reveals the social impact of conditions like diabetes on low-income populations who are largely overlooked in epidemiological transitions in low-income countries. Meena's narrative challenges the scholarly understanding of diabetes in India and illustrates that the experience of diabetes as an illness is fundamentally different when people face economic scarcity. This narrative reveals how the confluence of poverty, cultural change, social demands, psychological distress, and care-seeking delays create a unique syndemic within a context focused on social mobility and material success.

Chapter 4 centers on Sibongile's story from Soweto, a historic collection of six clustered townships in Johannesburg, South Africa. Sibongile faces complex intersections of structural violence produced by a legacy of apartheid and AIDS as well as personal insecurities in everyday life. Sibongile's narrative demonstrates the powerful role of cultural and political history in the emergent reality of diabetes, and it illustrates how lived experiences shape and are shaped by mental and physical health. For example, I unpack myriad forms of structural and interpersonal violence that become fundamental to the experience of illness. I also discuss how the social and financial demands placed on women who care for AIDS-orphaned grandchildren require more than love and money for school. In many cases women in Soweto, including Sibongile, prioritized the needs of their family members above their personal needs, including the need to manage their diet and medicines. Moreover, in a context of HIV stigma, Sibongile and others describe how diabetes becomes consumed in a catch-all chronic illness stigma whereby people conflate their diabetes treatment needs with those associated with HIV.

Chapter 5 unveils the complicated nature of Kandace's financial and personal insecurities at home and within the clinical sphere, which have resulted in unintended consequences for her diabetes. Like elsewhere, in Nairobi structural violence and poverty have a profound impact on how people eat, move, and interact. Personal insecurities also appear to be more profound in Nairobi when compared to all other study sites, as women with diabetes reported up to twelve co-occurring social stressors in their life stories. The social impact of AIDS, much like in Soweto, has played a fundamental role in transforming how people conceive of chronic illness and care seeking. Unlike in Soweto, however, people in Nairobi must pay out-of-pocket for diabetes care. This creates a clear financial divide between those who have health conditions for which treatment is free (HIV) and those who have conditions that require costly therapies (diabetes). This is one reason people exclaimed, "Diabetes is worse than HIV!"

In the conclusion I return to the simple argument that culture and experience fundamentally shape how diabetes is enacted cross-culturally. This chapter reflects on the four ethnographic case studies and proposes five ways in which anthropologists and public health practitioners should rethink diabetes. First, I argue that diabetes must be understood as a disease of poverty as opposed to exclusively one of modernization. Second, I argue that diabetes is always syndemic, especially when it confronts the complexities of economic insecurity. Third, diagnosis transforms how people perceive and experience their physical condition, revealing how knowing and naming a condition can have substantial social and emotional impact. Fourth, I suggest that the social life of diabetes contributes to fundamentally shifting what it means to have and live with diabetes across contexts. Finally, I argue that interventions for diabetes should employ syndemic thinking by working both upstream to address social policy and downstream to navigate clinical challenges and community-based solutions.

1

SYNDEMIC DIABETES

María

María's husband died from diabetes eight years before I met her. After fifty-eight years of living in Mexico, María left to visit her children in Chicago, where she planned to stay for less than a year. María stayed much longer, however, mostly caring for her grandson and working as a nanny. She lived for many years with her daughter and son-in-law. Even though she missed her siblings terribly, she never visited them because she was undocumented and feared she would not be able to return to visit her grandchildren in the United States if she left Chicago. When she arrived in Chicago in 2002 she also carried depression, hypertension, and diverticulitis across the border into her new life. In many ways, these things she carried with her haunted her memory and materialized in her body over several years, becoming reflected in her insulin resistance. After she settled into her new life, she found the grocery stores and medical care to be reason enough to stay.

María was dressed in a red sweatshirt and was bouncing to music on her iPod Nano when I met her. She carried the level of energy and look of a woman much younger than her sixty-five years. María's waist circumference of 49 inches, however, revealed extreme obesity. She associated her obesity with her depression, explaining, "Sometimes I feel too much sadness, too much like I want to cry. Then I tell my daughter, 'Geez, I can't cry, I don't get anything from when I cry.'" María's tears flowed from many events that marked her life story. Her father died when she was young, so, as the eldest of nine, María helped her mother raise her siblings, never attending school, until she left home at fifteen to marry. María explained, "We suffered a great deal of poverty and I know that my mother didn't want me. And I preferred to leave the house because a man, who wasn't my boyfriend, said nothing more than, 'Let's go.' And I went with him and we had many children." Marriage, however, did not solve her problems. María continued, "And later he left me. And he left me with eight children and I had to work to raise them. Later I met another man and we had one child together but he gave me a bad life. He hit me a lot, a lot, a lot. All my life I have suffered. And since he has died I have stayed alone here [in Chicago] with my children."

María was grateful for her eight years in the United States. She was most grateful to be there for her grandson, for whom she had cared since his birth, during a time of enormous upheaval in his life. After Thanksgiving dinner, María's son-in-law beat her seven-year-old grandson in front of her. María, who had experienced years of domestic abuse, found his actions unforgiveable. Having realized her daughter grieved but did nothing, María moved out of her daughter's home with her grandson and began supporting him by working as a nanny for a wealthy family in Chicago's northern suburbs. Financially independent for the first time in her life, María found a new freedom. She saved money, paid her own rent, and provided her grandson with a safe home.

Yet the complicated layers of stress in María's life caused her diverticulitis to act up. Two years before the interview, María came to the public hospital clinic with pain in her stomach. She left with a diabetes diagnosis, which spurred anxious memories of helping her late husband manage his diabetes with food and medicines that were insufficient and scarce. She did not associate diabetes with her childhood poverty, her abusive husband, or immigration experiences, as many women who participated in my research did. Instead, María associated her diabetes with *susto de dolor*—a fright that stemmed from the pain in her colon associated with her diverticulitis, not dissimilar from the deeply unsettling frights that many of the women in this study grieved. She connected her diabetes not only with this pain but also with fear of the disease associated with her husband's death. María explained:

> All he could have was juice with nopal, sábila—and I would make it. He'd ask me to put in pineapple, and I wouldn't put in pineapple. Later in the morning, then he would ask for an apple, banana, yogurt, and I would give it to him. He would want beans, I didn't give it. He would want tortilla, I wouldn't give it. And you know, I ate everything. I didn't care for myself. It was suicide for diabetes. . . . He died in September and I came [to Chicago] in October. He killed himself.

María's siblings wanted her to return to Mexico. However, María valued being close to her children in Chicago and caring for her grandson. She also valued the medical care she received at the public hospital clinic—something her husband could not access in Mexico, as he passed away many years before Seguro Popular, the political initiative that increased health care access for everyone beginning in the mid-2000s. Feeling socially isolated from her siblings posed a great emotional challenge, but María stayed. "I am very content and I am attended to medically," she noted. She explained that she feared returning to Mexico and having to pay for medical bills, especially for her diverticulitis: "These things cost a lot of money and I don't pay for them here. And I am very content." She went on to say, "But I don't sleep."

Syndemic Diabetes

María's narrative reveals how emotion, trauma, and distress materialize in her diabetes. The synergistic interaction of these social, psychological, and biological factors reveals a dynamic that is more complicated and integrative than any discrete measure of disease. It also reflects a more nuanced understanding of what drives her sickness and how she perceives and experiences illness. Yet, María's story can be imprinted onto a broader epidemiological narrative that elucidates how such factors travel together with population-level trends. In this case, it is the dual escalation of depression and diabetes among those of Mexican origin that, according to the narratives, cannot be dissociated from dynamics of immigration, financial insecurity, abuse, and social exclusion. Together, these social and health conditions comprise a syndemic.

A syndemic embodies the *syn*ergies of epi*demics*, whereby two or more conditions cluster together within a community, interact at the biological, psychological, or social level, and are driven by social or political factors.[1] For example, diabetes and depression cluster together within many communities that experience social or economic disadvantage[2]—and this relationship has been revealed in various studies in social epidemiology.[3] Yet, a core aspect of the syndemic production of diabetes and depression is their bidirectional biological and social interactions, which cannot be divorced from one another.[4] I will return to the two key features that make something syndemic—the disease-focused interactions and the epidemiological clustering—in what follows; here, I focus on the third attribute of syndemics: the role of social and political factors in driving the clustering and interaction of two or more diseases. The diabetes in María's life, therefore, represents a much broader collection of synergistic problems that travel together in her life, body, and community. These complex and dynamic interactions can be understood through her embodied suffering that reflects a broader syndemic.

Syndemic Suffering

The concept of syndemic suffering draws from two central theories in medical anthropology. First, syndemic suffering explicitly plays off of the fundamental theory of social suffering posed by Arthur Kleinman, Veena Das, and Margaret Lock (1997), which promoted the now widely accepted view that structural violence underlies poor health among socially and economically marginalized populations. First proposed by Johan Galtung (1969), the notion of structural violence suggests that structural (indirect) factors may be as powerful as physical (direct) factors in producing disease and suffering. Although theoretically invisible, structural violence becomes visible in the hegemony of institutions, ideologies, and inequalities that shape everyday lives (such as the market, trade, racist policies, economic isolation of some groups, and so on). Discrimination in the legal and social spheres, gender inequality, and racism also become visible forms of such violence. Linking the experience of the social world to violence, as Paul Farmer (1997a, 2001, 2004) has famously done,[5] reveals how powerful the hegemony of institutions, laws, and ideologies can be in shaping people's everyday lives, becoming reflected in the body and measured in the sickness of individuals and communities. Syndemic suffering addresses these historically deep and geographically broad[6] processes that shape individual suffering—while linking such processes to coalesced epidemiologies. For example, this became realized in María's life by way of her childhood deprivation and the resultant demands that she should forgo further schooling because her family needed her wages. Later in life, María's chronic illness was similarly materially structured as she struggled to purchase foods to manage her diabetes. Living in a food desert—where fresh foods were available but people were often priced out of eating a low-calorie, high-nutrient diet due to lack of affordability or access—played a pivotal role in her diabetes. As such, being socially located within a lower socioeconomic position since childhood shaped her life's chances and long-term health. It is important to note, however, that this did not stymie María's spirit or perseverance.

Second, the notion of syndemic suffering draws from critical phenomenology to consider how macro-social processes shape subjective experiences of temporalities, geographies, embodied suffering, social lives, and the self.[7] This reflects in part the critical phenomenology of Robert Desjarlais's *Sensory Biographies* (2003) and João Biehl's *Vita* (2005) and *Will to Live* (2007), because the intimate details of people's lives lay bare the structural inequalities that undergird them. I employ what Sarah Willen (2007, 12) has conceived as "phenomenologically sensitive portraits" to reveal how structural inequalities drive anxiety-ridden and frightening realities that stay in and move through the body. Doing so enables a critical interpretation of the black box of stress that is contingent to local realities as well as to individual and collective experiences of being-in-the-world.[8] Importantly, this approach shifts the perspective from the suffering of the patient to the experience of the sister, mother, caregiver, laborer, and citizen.

These intimate portraits reveal how violence can become manifest in more subtle ways. Bourdieu and Wacquant (2004) critique the concept of structural violence for limiting our focus on how social life can inflict extreme suffering, and instead they draw out the intimacies of symbolic and everyday (or normalized) violence. Symbolic violence addresses the visceral ways in which people perceive themselves to be socially dominated through sexism, racism, and classism. For instance, the cultural ideas about gender and power that contributed to María's perception that marriage was the only way to escape an abusive childhood exemplify symbolic violence. Whereas structural violence is empirically material, symbolic violence communicates culturally embedded vulnerabilities.

On the other hand, everyday violence refers to those repeated microaggressions that occur so frequently that they become routine, normalized experiences in everyday life.[9] These feelings of personal insecurity are exemplified in the hypervigilance that is so deeply felt when people walk through their neighborhood and feel unsafe or carry the threat of gun violence with them from school to their home. María may have carried a fear of the threat associated with being aggressively assaulted and deported by the police due to her undocumented status. María and others also relayed the deeply unsettling sense of normalization that afflicts the many women in this book who experienced sexual assault—for example, when feeling the threat of assault at home or encountering a perpetrator at a family gathering. It is impossible to disconnect these social and emotional pathways from biological risk. This complexity results from what Nancy Scheper-Hughes (1989, 14) called three decades ago the "real pathogens in this environment of high risk," such as poverty, deprivation, sexism, food insecurity, and economic exploitation.

The concept of fear brings these phenomenologies of violence into focus. Fear is a powerful accompaniment to the breakdown of social protection and the persistence of economic and personal insecurities that have become a way of life in the neoliberal era. Linda Green's ethnography of rural Guatemalan women reflects this, as she describes how fear and mistrust emerged amid decades of state oppression and civil war and how the "social relations of power, of gender, and of cultural production were shifting under the pressure of local economic insecurity perpetuated by larger structures of exploitation" (1999, 87). Whereas Green spoke of her interlocutors' oppression in the wake of conflict, the fear I speak of emanates explicitly from those less visible forms of violence that Philippe Bourgois (2009) calls "invisible." The fear discussed in the present study is not born from war; rather, it comes from structural violence that produces experiences of personal insecurity in the home and street, such as domestic violence and gun violence. In these cases, fear becomes realized through feeling unsafe, mistrust of other people (even neighbors), and expectations of struggle and hardship. This also includes the uncertainty of financial insecurity and of keeping one's family satisfied and safe. Such fears cannot be divorced from the particular historical set of economic, political, and cultural arrangements that produce social inequalities and hierarchies that subjugate women and create many spaces throughout their lives in which they feel unsafe.

Biological Underpinnings

What makes these complicated processes syndemic is in part the powerful biological processes that link structural and social inequalities with individual bodies. Envisioning María's story as a clinical case, one might emphasize her risk factors for diabetes such as her weight, ethnicity, age, high blood pressure, and potentially high cholesterol.[10] The risk factors perspective traditionally adopted by public health and clinical medicine discourse typically narrows down to focus on the most visible and discrete physical problems to the exclusion of the interactions among lingering memories, powerful emotions, and somatic responses that affect how María perceives and experiences diabetes. Yet, understanding the biology of diabetes provides the foundation for making sense of how trauma becomes embodied in (and therefore syndemic with) diabetes and depression.

At the most basic level, insulin is a hormone produced by the pancreas that is released into the blood stream to break down sugars. Those who develop insulin resistance cannot reduce sugar in the blood (known as blood glucose concentrations) to normal levels. Normally, the body breaks down carbohydrates (like tortillas, rice, bread, or other starches) into sugar for energy. Because those who are insulin resistant cannot break down these sugars, eating foods that carry less sugar is imperative for people with diabetes. Elevated glucose concentrations eventually contribute to organ damage (especially kidney failure), loss of sight, numbness in hands, and sores on feet. Many also experience episodes of heart attack and stroke. Taking medications such as metformin, which is the most common, or insulin injections enables the body to break down these sugars and prevents further diabetes disability. The slow way in which diabetes advances in the body, however, means that most people may not realize they are sick until complications arise. This is one reason more than half of those with type 2 diabetes are estimated to be undiagnosed and to receive a diagnosis only when a severe symptom or other problem drives them to seek medical care.[11]

Understanding the biological realities of those, like María, who face the compounded effects of chronic stress and acutely traumatic experiences requires a turn to the extensive literature on the psychophysiology of stress. In biology, stress is conceived as a threat to a stable state known as homeostasis. This threat involves three elements: the stressor that induces change in the body, the change (or disharmony) in the body, and the body's response to it.[12] The mind and the body work in mutual response to such stressors, and their response depends on the type, intensity, and duration of the stressor, or what is often called a stimulus (as well as the individual's state at the time in which the stress is experienced). In the case of stressors faced by women like María, such as many years of domestic violence, an acute stressor may become a chronic one. When stressors are severe and repetitive, the body does not react in its normal fight-or-flight response.[13] Instead, the body produces elevated amounts of glucocorticoids to bring the body back to normal and reduce inflammation. Cortisol is the most important glucocorticoid that regulates a variety of human functions; it is elevated in the body when people experience traumas such as domestic violence, racism (for instance, repeated in the workplace), or other forms of abuse, as well as structural inequalities that produce omnipresent stress, such as feeling unsafe in one's neighborhood.

We know from the Adverse Childhood Experiences (ACE) studies that childhood experiences, both positive and negative, can have an extraordinary impact on future violence victimization and perpetration as well as lifelong health.[14] ACEs incorporate not only instances of sexual, physical, or emotional abuse but also deeply influential social experiences from childhood, like stress related to parental violence, divorce, incarceration, or having a family member struggling with mental illness or substance abuse. When children experience multiple, overlapping conditions, their ACE score increases and they experience a "dose response"—which means that the more intense their childhood stress, the more likely they are to suffer from mental, physical, behavioral, or social problems later in life. For instance, longitudinal studies suggest that having experienced one ACE can escalate propensity for enduring psychological suffering, such as depression or alcoholism, as an adult. Having experienced two ACEs can increase one's likelihood of smoking, a practice many use to accommodate stress in their lives, and may be reflected in acute physical manifestations such as becoming severely obese or having a stroke. An ACE score of three adverse experiences during childhood has been associated in several large-scale studies with less physical activity and higher cardiometabolic distress, such as diabetes, stroke, heart disease.[15] Thus these studies carefully document how frequent exposure to acutely traumatic and prolonged stressful experiences may be linked with real, pathological, and subjectively painful biological changes.

An abundance of research on the psychophysiology of trauma indicates that such experiences are linked to depression and diabetes independently.[16] In a paper published in the *Lancet*, Moulton, Pickup, and Ismail (2015) describe how depression and diabetes "share biological origins, particularly overactivation of innate immunity leading to a cytokine-mediated inflammatory response, and potentially through dysregulation of the hypothalamic-pituitary-adrenal axis" (from which elevated cortisol release stems).[17] Moreover, as a result of feeling stressed or depressed, people move less and crave oily, salty, and sweet foods. When people are severely depressed and medicated for their depression, they are also more prone to gain weight. Notably, the social and structural factors that undergird these interactions have real and visible costs. The most consequential are the need for dialysis, amputation, and blindness—and the most severe is death. These physical realities manifest quickly among those who delay seeking care. Most delay seeking care for flagship symptoms—like elevated thirst or numbness in the extremities—due to high costs or a lack of familiarity with what these symptoms might signal.

These biological underpinnings are in part what makes the interaction of social traumas, poverty, fear, diabetes, and depression syndemic. This process is intimately linked to stress hormones like cortisol that make cells more likely to become insulin resistant in the first place. When blood sugar drops (due to insulin), people feel hungry. If individuals are insulin resistant, however, the brain does not direct them to stop eating (by making them feel full), so they are more likely to want to continue eating. This is because the body wants to store fat.[18] This is insulin working *through* the hypothalamus—the part of the brain that communicates thirst, hunger, sleepiness, emotion, and body temperature.[19] This is exacerbated further by the stress hormone cortisol, which increases exponentially within the body when our social worlds create physical chaos.[20] Cortisol is an important link, as it acts on fat cells throughout the body to make them more insulin resistant. Thus, increased and persistent stress (measured by cortisol release as well as elevated baseline levels) makes one feel hungrier, crave sugar, and gain weight.[21] All this has been tested and scrutinized in multiple longitudinal studies, revealing that life events, sleeping problems, anger, and hostility—measured in social distress and chronic depression—increase risk for diabetes.[22] Perhaps, however, they are most easily understood in María's story, which weaves together childhood poverty, the loss of her father at a young age, spousal abuse, her husband's chronic illness, and finally her own illness. The combined chronic stressors and traumatic experiences revealed in her narrative no doubt contributed to her round middle, depression, and diabetes.

Many convincing hypotheses about the relationship between stress and diabetes come from the Developmental Origins of Health and Disease (DOHaD) studies.[23] DOHaD scientists are concerned with what David Barker (1995, 1999) proposed to be the developmental (or fetal) origins hypothesis. Barker insisted that babies who were born small because of nutritional stress were more likely to develop chronic diseases later in life when compared to babies born at healthier birth weights.[24] Based on numerous physiological facts that link low birth weight with adult obesity and diabetes,[25] this theory prioritized social and economic conditions that cause stress as the root of the unequal distribution of chronic diseases among the population.[26] These were some of the earliest studies of epigenetics, which is a field of study that reveals how the environment can transform gene expression, modifying individuals' risk for some diseases simply based on their interactions in the world.[27]

Anthropologists have contributed significantly to this scholarship, demonstrating how epigenetic pathways—which show how the environment gets into the genes—contribute to cardiovascular and metabolic disease inequalities.[28] The biological anthropologists Zaneta Thayer and

Amy Non (2015, 723) explain: "An understanding of epigenetics suggests that it is not just the genes with which you are born but also the environment into which you are born that appears to be important for predicting your health or disease risk." Some scholars contend that such epigenetic changes are passed on over generations.[29] A number of cohort studies in low- and middle-income countries have confirmed the social origin of prematurity and low birth weight, stressing the influence of poverty and nutritional stress in utero and during the first years of life.[30] Yet other anthropologists, such as Emily Yates-Doerr (2015, 45), warn that one must be wary of "teleological frameworks in which a cause at one point in time leads to the determinant effect in another," because political, social, and economic contexts shift and move through time. Nevertheless, this scholarship underscores the powerful link between the body and the environment—a link that is moving through time and space in meaningful, nonlinear pathways.

Finally, it is worthy to note that a growing body of biomedical research takes seriously how social and ecological factors may become realized through epigenetic processes in diabetes. An article in the prestigious medical journal *Nature* written by Christian Fuchsberger and colleagues (2016) in collaboration with 300 scientists argued that the environment plays a pivotal role in diabetes.[31] For instance, the authors maintain that the environment, and its interaction with genes, has greater influence on diabetes risk than genes alone. They also stated that genetics does not explain population differences with regard to who has increased risk for diabetes, suggesting that the hypotheses that some populations are genetically susceptible to diabetes are misled. This notion reflects Michael Montoya's (2007) argument that the "bioethical conscription" of risk, which attributes risk to ethnicity, may obfuscate historical and structural subjugation that can play out in epigenetic realities. The authors further unpack a biological process whereby environmental factors can influence the beta cells involved in insulin resistance in order to spur diabetes, revealing one path through which stress causes diabetes. Finally, they suggest that more longitudinal research that takes seriously the complex ways through which environments get under the skin is imperative.[32] Although their notion of environment still remains somewhat underdeveloped, there is promise in the increasing recognition of the immense role of social and ecological factors in the production of diabetes. Indeed, these interactions are what make it syndemic.

Clustering

The focus of syndemics on the social and corporeal worlds puts them apart from clinical notions of comorbidity or multimorbidity. However, its emphasis on what, how, and where two or more conditions cluster together is what puts syndemic theory apart also from other prevailing epidemiological scholarship on the social determinants of health. The focus on what diseases cluster together within a population or a geographic space is exactly what brings medical anthropological thinking into the fields of social epidemiology, public health, and clinical medicine. In fact, Merrill Singer and Scott Clair (2003) made this convincingly clear early on in the construction of the syndemic approach. In what follows, I discuss how to think about what diseases cluster together, where they materialize, and who is most affected.

The theory of syndemics reflects the work of Michael Marmot, Geoffrey Rose, and others who in the 1970s and 1980s explored social stratification and health inequalities in the United Kingdom through what are known as the Whitehall Studies. This scholarship inspired a generation of investigators to interrogate why poverty makes people sick and directed the large body of scholarship on the social determinants of health.[33] For instance, Nancy Krieger's (1994, 2001) pioneering work on ecosocial theories considers how biological, social, and ecological systems become embodied and manifest in poor health.[34] Jo Phelan, Bruce Link, and others' (2004, 2010) theory of fundamental causes makes clear how social and political forces drive concentrated health disparities. Lisa Berkman and Ichiro Kawachi (2000) demonstrate how society and social organizations influence health and well-being. What syndemics contribute to this literature is a clear understanding of what social and economic factors drive clustered epidemics, which have clear bio-psycho-social interactions, and how such clusters may produce a negative feedback loop to further complicate social and medical conditions at once.

A first defining characteristic of a syndemic is that two or more conditions must cluster together within a certain population, causing more sickness than any social or health condition would alone.[35] The epidemiological data available for diabetes, HIV, tuberculosis, and depression in India, Kenya, South Africa, and the United States is imperfect, but when systematically organized, the data tell an important story about the complexity of syndemic diabetes in urban enclaves.[36] Table 3 shows how these conditions cluster together among low-income people in these urban enclaves and reveals how risk for diabetes, HIV, tuberculosis, and depression is comparably higher among these communities compared to the population at large.[37] Whenever possible, table 3 draws data from studies focused on Chicago, Delhi, Johannesburg/Soweto, and Nairobi/Kibera. Recognizing these geographic vulnerabilities is an imperative step before unpacking how and why inequalities perpetuate syndemics, because it illustrates what conditions co-occur among these populations.

TABLE 3. Estimated Prevalence by Country and Urban Poor[38]

	Diabetes	Depression	HIV/AIDS	Tuberculosis
India				
Population	8.6%–15.5%	4.5%–15%	0.31%	0.2%–0.4%
Urban poor	11%–12%	19.3%	0.35%	0.46%–1.1%
Kenya				
Population	3.6%	7%–66%	6%	0.3%
Urban poor	4.8%–10%	30%	10.6%–12%	0.7%[i]
South Africa				
Population	7.1%–8.3%	5%–10%	11%–20%	0.8%
Urban poor	12.1%	9%	22%–30%	1%–5.5%
United States				
Population	9%–11%	6.6%	0.4%–0.9%	0%
Urban poor	10%–14%	15.4%	2.1%	0.97%[ii]

i These are cause-of-death data for urban slum populations.
ii These data are from New York City only.

This table's overlap of diabetes with depression matters because depression not only is the most common co-occurring condition with diabetes,[39] but it also deeply and unevenly afflicts the social lives of women. Increasingly, scholars have unpacked the depression-diabetes paradigm, demonstrating a bidirectional relationship[40] and showing that economic hardship further increases the risk of concurrent depression in diabetes.[41]

This is a powerful relationship because, on the one hand, mental illness often goes undetected, and on the other hand, mental distress can severely undermine daily life.

Moreover, an increasing number of studies are documenting the biological and social interactions of diabetes with HIV and with tuberculosis. Such interactions become syndemic because they are connected to important social and economic features. For instance, the convergence of diabetes and HIV[42] is associated with the availability of effective ART, which has increased the longevity of those living with HIV by a decade.[43] This is further complicated by the long-established relation of HIV with mental illness and structural inequalities, with depression and food insecurity posing an extraordinary risk to individuals living with HIV disease.[44] Similarly, living in areas affected by high rates of pulmonary tuberculosis, including multidrug-resistant and extensively drug-resistant tuberculosis (MDRTB and XDRTB, respectively), poses enhanced complexity and risk of diabetes.[45] Tuberculosis-diabetes interactions have received increasing international attention,[46] in part because diabetes unidirectionally triples the risk for active tuberculosis.[47] The complex social and structural risks that produce the conditions for these diseases to become syndemic reveal how biological and medical remedies may fall short in addressing environmental risk, and they underscore the importance of implicating non-medical features when evaluating "risk" for disease and "compliance" of treatment.

These epidemiological and biological data question not only the interworking of disease convergence but also the social lives of those who experience them. Recognizing how cramped urban spaces might concurrently impede physical activity and promote obesity, increase feelings of personal insecurity and the distress associated with them, and expose one to the *mycobacterium tuberculosis* is fundamental for unpacking the syndemic underpinnings of emergent and persistent problems. Through this prism of clustering complexity, then, we can realize how the social traumas and chronic poverty experienced throughout the life course interconnect with such physical and psychological marks, demanding that we move from biology to social life.

The Biosocial Production of Risk

Syndemic theory moves beyond looking exclusively to the clustering of co-occurring conditions because it takes seriously the biosocial production of disease within and between populations. In his earliest work on the syndemics of HIV and AIDS, Merrill Singer brought into focus the social construction, social transmission, and social location of disease, examining these social dimensions alongside the structural inequalities that give them shape. Singer (1994) argued that AIDS is a human experience (1) socially located along society's "fault lines";[48] (2) socially transmitted through human behaviors and the politics and power that shape risk; and (3) socially constructed by way of social definitions, values, and relationships. Ron Stall and colleagues have furthered this type of syndemic thinking by deconstructing the role of the social in constructing risk, or what they call "syndemic production."[49] In what follows, I discuss these foundational ideas.

First, the concept of fault lines has been employed by medical anthropologists to describe how inequalities converge with emotion, disease, and suffering within particular social contexts and phenomena, from fear to infectious diseases and illicit drugs;[50] therefore, this notion provides a fundamental heuristic for syndemic theory. Like AIDS, diabetes appears to "move along the fault lines of society"[51] as it clusters among low-income populations in high- and low-income countries alike. Such alignments of deprivation have been described elsewhere as "clusters of disadvantage"[52] or "hot spots"[53] in medicine, indicating that it is possible to essentially map where social and medical problems cluster together. These fault lines have also been articulated as "risk environments" that, according to Rhodes and colleagues, require one to focus on "the *social situations, structures,* and *places* in which risk is produced" (2005, 1027; original emphasis) as opposed to blaming the victim by placing the onus of risk on individuals' behaviors and relationships. In this way, fault lines structure how social and health problems are aligned epidemiologically because clusters of disadvantage show "how multiple features of risk and inequality intersect to produce geographical vulnerability" (2005, 1030).

Income inequality plays a fundamental role in creating fault lines in the contexts discussed in this book. In their classic report "Wider income gaps, wider waistbands?" Kate Pickett and colleagues (2005, 670) argue that the "psychosocial stress of life near the bottom of a steeply hierarchical society is a suggested explanation for [the] associations" between income inequality and negative health effects, including diabetes and its complications. It is the confluence of gendered subjectivities, persistent financial insecurities, and social problems that accompanies economic deprivation in unequal and hierarchal societies and provokes psychosocial stress. The intimacy of these experiences, as it is revealed through narratives, is rarely captured in social determinants of health frameworks or ecosocial models that aim to unpack how economic inequalities get under the skin. However, it is exactly the entanglement of social problems at the bottom of the social ladder that perpetuates the suffering linked to diabetes, depression, and their overlap. These challenges are exemplified by the trade-offs many families make every day between paying for medical bills or paying for their children's school fees. Others make explicit choices about what foods they will feed their families based on cost, often privileging cheaper filler calories such as processed carbohydrates. In this way, income inequalities and health inequalities go hand-in-hand, revealing the importance of the fault line of economic deprivation for understanding the disproportionate health burden among the poor.

The second point made by Singer, concerning how disease is socially transmitted through human behaviors and the politics and power that shape risk, echoes the theory of local biologies employed by Margaret Lock (1993, 2001), and others. Lock (2001, 483) has argued that the theory of local biologies posits how evolutionary, environmental, and individual variables reflect an "embodied experience of physical sensations" that incorporates social, emotional, and biological reflections. This approach takes seriously how shared exposures and shared experiences among people attenuate the geographies of risk that structure syndemic suffering. This is why the definition of "risk" for diabetes must be locally interpreted; structural inequalities may shape the consumption of foods (public sphere) and pharmaceuticals (clinical sphere), while social dynamics produce intimate social-biological, social-psychological, and psychological-biological interactions. Esther's story provides an example: On the one hand, in Kenya the pervasiveness of AIDS affects how Esther perceives diabetes not only socially but also biologically, linking the two diseases together in her conception of what diabetes is. On the other hand, her experiences living with HIV and seeking treatment for it play a role in her diabetes diagnosis and in her juxtaposition of diabetes care and routine medical care for HIV. Hence, diabetes itself is socially produced through local notions of sickness through which people define suffering and model care-seeking. Thus, adapting one intervention for diabetes from one context where HIV prevalence is low may not be effective in another context where HIV prevalence is very high.

This is why understanding the concepts of diabetes "risk" and "compliance" is imperative. Anthropology's conception of risk contrasts sharply with that of biomedical sciences and public health. Anthropologists often conceive risk to be situated within broader social and structural frameworks that shape how people move in the world.[54] In contrast, biomedicine and public health speak of risk in terms of discrete markers and individual behaviors and interventions. Mark Nichter (2008) argues that the concept of risk is, in and of itself, a product of the culture of biomedicine that overlooks the structural undercurrents of behaviors such as eating, moving, and caring for one's health. Clinical expectations may pose dilemmas to the patients. Hearing what one must do for diabetes care is one thing; recognizing the inconceivability of what that self-care demands in the face of competing social, financial, and family demands is another. When rethinking diabetes, we must recognize how the differential risk associated with residing in resource-poor settings fundamentally transforms the experience of diabetes for some.

It is critical to unpack the risk environments that make the two essential components of diabetes control for the biomedical model—diet and exercise—terribly difficult to accomplish. For instance, low-income communities often reside in food deserts defined by the lack of supermarkets and the invasive presence of a plethora of corner stores and fast-food chains that offer easy access to energy-dense (or empty-calorie) foods. This causes many families to consume processed foods that are high in fat, sugar, and salt, leading to more obesity and diabetes.[55] However, because the concept of the food desert was based on the experience of wealthy nations like the United States, the notion does not easily translate across geopolitical contexts. For example, in Kenya fast food chains target the wealthy as opposed to the poor. Moreover, many low-income urban Indians and South Africans have ample opportunities to buy fresh foods, but they may opt to consume cheap processed foods, sugar-sweetened beverages, or fried snacks because of affordability and ease.[56] Low-income neighborhoods in both Chicago and Nairobi may both be defined as food deserts, even though the concept of the food *desert* may appear even more appropriate in Kibera due to the structural impediments to purchase fresh fruits and vegetables, as their costs have steeply increased following swift economic change. Although the degree and the type of structural, cultural, and personal challenges vary across individuals and geographies of vulnerability, what is universal is that the confluence of these factors makes the personal responsibility to manage one's diet stressful. Recognizing the local divergences, however, matters when thinking about syndemically driven interventions.

In conclusion, rethinking diabetes syndemically requires that we understand how multiple latitudes of suffering become visible within the body, are enacted in lived lives, and materialize within and between communities. I end this section with a final comment on health conditions, especially HIV and tuberculosis, that converge with diabetes in the pages to follow. Lenore Manderson and Carolyn Smith-Morris (2010) have wisely cautioned that we must move beyond the chronic/acute distinctions that so commonly place noncommunicable and infectious conditions in disparate categories of meaning. They argue in *Chronic Conditions, Fluid States* that the binaries of communicable/noncommunicable and acute/chronic are social facts but not social realities:

> The distinction of chronic-acute is inaccurate even in biomedical terms, since the notion of acute fails to distinguish between: (a) conditions that are relatively benign and self-limiting; (b) those that are life threatening; and (c) those that shift from an acutely symptomatic phase to an extended period of poor health and physical limitations, as is characteristic of numerous medical conditions that have effective medicinal or therapeutic treatments. (Manderson and Smith-Morris 2010, 3–4)

They contend therefore that the experience of an illness matters more than the cause. People with HIV are now living decades longer than years past, and complicated challenges such as going hungry, feeling isolated, struggling with treatments, and suffering from co-infections will only become more complicated with conditions like diabetes. Thinking through how and where diabetes becomes syndemic with HIV is becoming one of the greatest challenges in global health for the coming decades. The pages to follow provide some insight into how people experience, perceive, and care for such convergence.

2

CHICAGO

Beatriz

Slouched over a magazine in the General Medicine Clinic (GMC) of the largest public hospital in Chicago, Beatriz passed the time waiting to meet with her doctor. She was seeking routine medical care for diabetes when we met. I approached Beatriz and apologized for interrupting her reading; she smiled and invited me to sit down. We chatted about the lengthy time she generally must wait for medical care at the clinic and the frequency with which she attended the clinic for her diabetes care. Because I had spent many hours in the GMC recruiting patients to participate in consecutive studies, Beatriz recognized me from her previous visits and became curious about my research when I mentioned it was a study of stress and diabetes.

Beatriz described a bicultural childhood; she was born in El Paso, Texas, and frequently crossed the border into Ciudad Juarez, where her grandmother lived. She maintained a close relationship with her grandmother

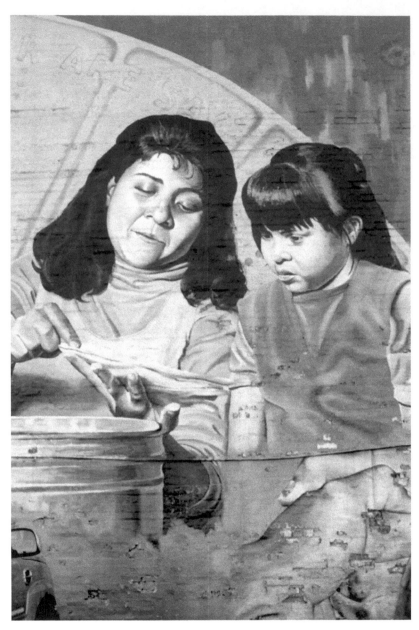

Figure 1. Mural in the Pilsen neighborhood.
Photo by Meredith Zielke.

in Juarez, but her domestic life in El Paso was strained after her father abandoned the family. Beatriz's mother became very abusive toward her; as Beatriz explained, "Every time she had a chance, she'd tell me she hates me—that I have the blood of my father." She explained that her mother's verbal abuse, which was often coupled with physical battering, caused her to leave home to marry at seventeen years of age. She soon became a mother and had four children with her first husband, before she left him because of his drinking and related physical abuse. She explained, "I don't know what's wrong with him. One day he pushed me against the wall [with his boot] and my head opened, like, this big [gesturing to indicate the gash in her head]." It was at this point that Beatriz decided to leave her husband. She married again, for a short period, and had two more children before she left her second husband for similar grievances of physical violence.

In her third marriage, Beatriz found her life partner, with whom she spent more than twenty-eight years and raised two more children (for a total of eight children in their household). Beatriz and her husband were employed in stable jobs in the service industry throughout their adult lives. However, their jobs were not well paid, and therefore they struggled to support their large family, living just above the poverty line. They had food on the table but limited expendable income. In addition, because of social factors in and around their neighborhood in Chicago—drug use, gang presence, educational barriers, job precarity, and persistent gun violence—Beatriz faced further challenges in supporting her children's futures. Some of these experiences touched her family in ways Beatriz could have never imagined, causing her deep pain and mental distress. These experiences were central to how she viewed the world and understood her own health and well-being

Beatriz's son was shot in December, a few years before my interview with her, during gang-related activity in her neighborhood. He was injured so severely that he was expected to die. Beatriz's grief was so intense that she attempted to commit suicide by overdosing on sleeping pills and was admitted to the psychiatric unit of an urban hospital for thirty-two days. She called this episode "going blank" and associated her hospitalization with the onset of diabetes. She said, "[It was the] stress that I created with that shooting of my son that got me diabetic."

Beatriz went on to explain: "After I lost the memory, they [in the psychiatric unit] almost kept me sleepy because they didn't want me to go back to that stage [of grief]. So they were feeding me, and I was going to bed, and feeding, and I gained up to 300 pounds. Right now I can say that I am skinny. [Laughter] And I'm still like, 215, 214 [pounds] I think." Weight gain is not uncommon for people who take antipsychotic medications like the ones Beatriz was most likely receiving during her hospitalization. Beatriz was diagnosed with diabetes four months later, when she returned to the hospital as a result of a work accident. She said, "They asked me how long I was a diabetic and I said, 'I'm not a diabetic.' The doctor said, 'Yes you have diabetes.'"

Beatriz's stress, however, did not end with her son's incident. She went on to explain, "My baby of the boys, Arturo, he was killed in a crossfire, too." I quietly asked her, "So you've lost two boys?" She replied, "No, the first one—he's alive, but he's in a wheelchair. But Artie [pause] was the lucky one. I don't know how to see it. But my son died [he did not live] to fifteen [years old]. Some guys were shooting and my little boy was cut through the window by a crazy bullet." Beatriz fell into her hands sobbing. Between cries she added, "It's been very hard for me."

Beatriz connected these two incidents not only because they were both related to gun violence but also because of her own responses to them. She went on, "I didn't lose my memory at that time, but I went crazy because I have a lot of [stress] at the present moment. Because of the other—what happened with my other son." In fact, her older son, who was still recuperating from his shooting at the time, fell into drinking and other drugs following the loss of his brother. Since then, Beatriz has been taking 300 mg of bupropion (also known as Wellbutrin), a depression medication, daily. Beatriz commented, "I had a lot of counseling and the counseling helps you, but you don't forget the situation, right? You just cope with it, you know. You just learn how to live with it."

Like many women I interviewed, Beatriz linked the stress of her life with her physical and psychological illness and suffering. In the years after her son's death, Beatriz developed physical pain that was difficult to overcome through massage, rest, or other treatments. After numerous doctor visits, including an erroneous diagnosis of multiple sclerosis (MS),[1] her doctor settled with the diagnosis of fibromyalgia. Fibromyalgia is a biomedical term for widespread musculoskeletal pain, often accompanied by exhaustion, memory loss, and mood swings or alterations, which has no clear cause or origin. Beatriz explained:

> I just know that I was in a lot of pain. And I think they [the doctors] think [my fibromyalgia] was a psychological thing because they blame it on my depression. [Pause] They said that it was a stress, even my doctor said, well, it's what you are going through. . . . One day I felt even my heart tighten and I went to see the doctor again after two days and she told me that it was my depression, my stress, when I was feeling those pains. And at the same time I was taking Lipitor [a lipid lowering medication], samples of Lipitor, for my cholesterol.

Despite the personal and health problems in her life, Beatriz described financial insecurity as one of the key stressors, underscoring the strong interconnections between her poverty and her health. Beatriz explained, "The worst part happening right now is that I'm trying to get my house [mortgage refinanced] or we're gonna lose it. [Pause] It's been difficult for us, especially with my medicines. I spend [out of pocket] like $400 with medicines every two months." Because most of the women in my study lived well below the poverty line, I had not anticipated the fact that Beatriz's income status would make her ineligible for Medicaid.[2] I asked if she received her medicines through the county hospital system where she had currently come to seek diabetes care. Beatriz explained, "No, I don't [regularly] come here because I have insurance. My husband has insurance at work. In the private [insurance plan], the doctor gave me two [prescriptions for medicines] every month. But if I have to buy it, it was out of my pocket. 'Cause the insurance doesn't pay for it. It costs $250. That's what it costs and they don't cover it."

Methods and Context

I collected the narratives of Beatriz and other women in Chicago, a diverse metropolis with one in five people (around one million) reporting Mexican heritage. More than half of the one million people of Mexican descent reside in Chicago itself, with many claiming multiple generations of family history in Chicago. These "Mexicans" come from a broad spectrum of Mexican states, different ethnicities, and varied educational backgrounds, and many—though not all—maintain deep connections and everyday relations with various sending communities in Mexico.[3] The historical legacy of what many scholars have called Mexican Chicago reveals a rich intercultural space characterized by intimate, transgenerational ties with Mexico and ethnic discrimination and economic marginalization within Chicago itself.[4] The cultural complexities of what defines a Mexican identity in Chicago reveal how one ethnicity can be so multifaceted. Many are first-generation immigrants, including some who arrived during adolescence or early adulthood from Mexico or other areas of the United States, whereas others are second-, third-, or fourth-generation immigrants with strong community ties and cultural identities rooted in Mexican enclaves and in other mixed ethnic neighborhoods in Chicago and the surrounding suburbs.

Beatriz is one of 121 women I interviewed in the GMC at the John H. Stroger Jr. Hospital of Cook County, often referred to as the "new" Cook County Hospital (because it was built to replace the old, infamous public hospital). I spent four years conducting research in this clinic on various projects linked to immigration, culture, and diabetes.[5] Two in three women who shared their life stories with me were born in Mexico and had lived in Chicago more than 25 years and had settled in one of Chicago's Mexican enclaves such as Pilsen or La Villita (Little Village). Few of these women ever held jobs independent of the work they did for their families, and most lived with their children or in an apartment adjacent to one or more family members. Caregiving for family members—grandchildren, children, and neighbors, sometimes for pay—was often a part-time or full-time job. Many (though not all) of these women comprised the one quarter of my interlocutors who were undocumented. They shared diverse upbringings, with some having spent much of their childhoods living between border towns, such as Laredo, Texas, and Nuevo Laredo, Mexico. Many women crossed family and national borders with ease and led largely transnational, bicultural lives. Other women had spent much of their lives in Mexico, immigrating to Chicago only five to ten years before I met them to work as caregivers for their grandchildren or to seek comfort on the death of a husband. Others had never left Chicago's city limits. There was similar linguistic diversity, with roughly half of the women speaking Spanish only and the other half speaking both Spanish and English, with a handful speaking only English. Many had completed high school or more and had worked outside the home most of their adult lives, although many were retired or on disability due to poor health. Most of these women lived with their partners or on their own in apartments in ethnically diverse neighborhoods such as South Chicago and Logan Square.

This project examines the experiences of some of the poorest Mexicans in the city, unveiling how Chicago is a microcosm of the inequality that has strengthened its grip as it widens in the United States. Beatriz and others routinely received medical care at the GMC because few had insurance and most were living below or near to the poverty line.[6] They came to the GMC because there were few other places where they could seek medical care, and many described how thankful they were for the care they received. This was despite the multiple hours many waited to see their doctors and then the additive hours they spent waiting for medications at the overcrowded pharmacy in the same building.[7] In fact, Beatriz exemplifies the story of the nearly one in four Mexicans in Chicago who resided at or below the poverty line according to the 2000 census. Beatriz's family was in a quandary because, although she and her husband worked more than forty hours per week in multiple jobs, they could barely make ends meet in one of the United States' most prominent cities. Like many in the United States, Beatriz suffered a medical bankruptcy that ruined her financial security and threatened to make her homeless. Many others in the study reported similar financial situations, hovering below the extreme poverty line of $10,000 per year. Their experiences resemble those of many who reside on the margins of the most segregated cities in the United States, with persistent social and health disparities linked to residential neighborhoods.[8]

At the GMC, it was not difficult to identify and invite Mexican immigrant women with diabetes to speak with me. Diabetes is the seventh leading cause of death in the United States,[9] most frequently afflicting women who face structural violence, enduring poverty, and the repeated social traumas that are so common to urban enclaves. It is not surprising that depression partners so closely with diabetes among women pushed to the economic and social margins of society, and that it often goes untreated.

When I approached women at the clinic, most were friendly and eagerly agreed to spend a few hours speaking with me. This was because they expected to spend a number of hours waiting to meet with the doctors, and the nurses often were agreeable and managed to shift around women's appointments so they could speak with me in a private room. I think that some of the women participated in the interviews because they were compensated for their time, which is customary for research at the GMC.[10] Most women were pleased to have someone with whom to pass the time and found our conversations cathartic. One woman described our five hours together by these words: "I feel like I just had a therapy session!"[11] We spoke extensively about their lives and the most significant memories that sat at the tip of their tongues; I also collected finger-stick blood samples to analyze concentrations of glucose (sugar) in the blood,[12] various surveys on their diabetes, psychiatric inventories for depression[13] and post-traumatic stress disorder (PTSD),[14] and various anthropometrics.[15]

Beatriz's story was not unlike many other women's complicated and overlapping life events. Most were at least forty years of age but no older than sixty-five. All but two were married at some point in their lives, with children and bicultural families with children residing in various locations in Mexico and the United States. Every woman had lived with type 2 diabetes for at least a year, and on average the women had had diabetes for at least ten years. One in two women reported symptoms of depression according to a common measure for depression, and one in three reported depressive symptoms according to a very stringent measure. Forty percent reported PTSD symptoms. Most described their distress through cultural idioms such as *coraje* (described as a deep-seated rage). Somatic symptoms of distress were just as common, including chronic pain often in the lower back, head, and shoulders. Menopause was also commonly mentioned as a convergent social and biological reality.

I scrutinized each life history narrative to understand how women described stress and what stressors took hold in their everyday lives. This involved extensive memory work as women were telling their stories (as opposed to compiling a standard checklist), in some cases going back to their early childhoods. Although some stressors may have been left out, the experiences they did describe were undoubtedly the ones that had had the strongest impact on their lives. On average, women described three significant stressors, and in some cases specific stresses were strongly associated with checklists for symptoms of depression, PTSD, or physical distress. Figure 2 shows the major stressors and conveys the complexity of suffering that women like Beatriz described. Two-thirds reported interpersonal abuse, with physical abuse (54 percent) and sexual abuse (23 percent) being extremely common. Many of these experiences were from childhood and first marriages (often when they were teenagers). Some traumatic experiences were associated with immigration or the less

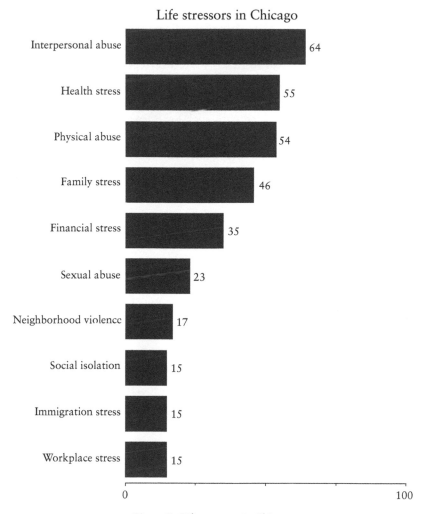

Figure 2. Life stressors in Chicago

visible social and emotional consequences of being undocumented. More than half of the women reported some physical health–related stress, and just under half reported family stress. One in three women reported financial insecurity as a stressor, and one in six women described neighborhood violence, immigration, work, and feelings of social isolation as sources of stress.

What is unique about this set of narratives is that they were collected together with multiple forms of data (biological, demographic, psychiatric) and evaluated inductively before they were transformed into deductive analyses. Quantitative analyses of these data revealed that those who reported any abuse, physical abuse, sexual abuse, social isolation, health stress, and diabetes distress were more likely to report symptoms of psychological distress (depression and in many cases PTSD).[16] Other stressors were not significantly linked to psychiatric measures, but in many ways they were intimately embedded with such experiences in women's narratives. Such analyses became a central organizing principle for the development of what I called the VIDDA syndemic—illustrating the close links between violence, immigration and isolation, depression, diabetes, and abuse.[17]

Syndemic Suffering in Chicago

In *Syndemic Suffering* (Mendenhall 2012), I first introduced the VIDDA syndemic, which deconstructs how violence, immigration, depression, diabetes, and abuse come together to frame sickness among low-income Mexican immigrant women in Chicago and underscores how these mutually interacting factors become entangled in broader frameworks (see figure 3).[18] For instance, Beatriz did not just suffer from diabetes; her suffering was syndemic through the interaction of social problems, economic insecurity, psychological distress, and other physical problems. Such experiences cannot be dissociated from the structural violence defined by a particular historical set of economic, political, and cultural arrangements within twenty-first-century capitalism that is embedded in social institutions and social relations. For example, subjugation along gender, class, and racial lines within Chicago has fueled rising home prices, declining incomes, and gentrifying neighborhoods. It has orchestrated food

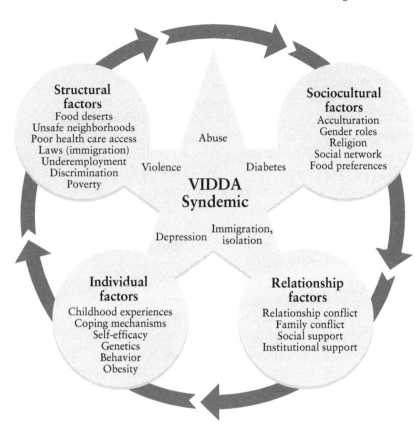

Figure 3. VIDDA syndemic

deserts that have cultivated hidden hungers. Violence within the city has escalated, as shown by the extraordinary rate of Chicago homicides. This has created the conditions for a deep-seated sense of insecurity among some. A unique form of discrimination connected to Mexican identity fosters both liminality as immigrants teeter between two worlds and a hierarchy of belonging between old and new immigrant families. All of these experiences are embodied in the health disparities that plague the urban poor in the United States, which are measurably higher than in most other industrialized nations.

The complex interactions within the VIDDA syndemic became clear in Beatriz's life story. Beatriz hints to a difficult childhood by mentioning the social exclusion she experienced as a child separated emotionally from her parents and physically from her grandmother (across a somewhat porous border). Leaving her family's home in her youth to get married was a somewhat risky move, although many women chose this path to escape difficult childhoods. Like Beatriz, however, many women found themselves in difficult marriages with varying levels of abuse or subjugation due to the unequal power dynamics within their new homes. Beatriz's strength to leave her first two marriages demonstrates that she overcame not only an arduous period of her life but also the difficult odds of escaping an abusive union. She described a happy marriage with her last partner as well as a tight-knit family. The grief she faced during adulthood is often overlooked in studies of women's health; the most traumatic and visceral experience from her adulthood was the injury of one son and the loss of another to crossfire. This social trauma effectively disabled her with grief, driving her into a medical journey that led to diabetes. This experience illuminates how family stress can become dissociated in the mind and communicated through the body. These experiences are then compounded by the chronicities of living with depression, diabetes, fibromyalgia, and other co-occurring conditions. Finally, Beatriz's financial insecurity put her between a rock and a hard place: at the time of her diabetes diagnosis she was not eligible for Medicaid, which put her family's livelihood in danger. When these chronic structural and social problems became convergent with chronic medical problems, her family fell deeper into the poverty that had fueled much of her distress in the first place.

Thus, the VIDDA syndemic conceptualizes five core factors that become realized syndemically in the lives of the Mexican women in Chicago I interviewed. First, *violence* encompasses structural, symbolic, and everyday forms. Second, *immigration*-related stress results from the experience of migration, the fear of deportation once arrived in the United States, and the feeling of social isolation that follows the loss of existing social networks. Third, *depression* is a chronic disorder for which very few poor women in the United States receive treatment, and which in many cases is prolonged and internalized for decades. Fourth, *diabetes* is what unites the women in this study, who also have myriad concurrent illnesses (insulin resistance both fuels and responds to the breakdown of the body). Finally, interpersonal *abuse* encompasses the salience of verbal, emotional, physical, and sexual abuse in women's life stories. These interlocking aspects of oppression help shape my interpretations of what it means to have diabetes in Chicago, and what this physical manifestation of stress may reveal about social experience. The rest of this chapter draws from multiple women's stories to depict VIDDA and the complex interactions within it.

Immigration, Poverty, and Abuse

What is evident from these women's narratives are the macro-level political, economic, and social inequalities that facilitate micro-level stresses. For example, financial stress and the breakdown of social networks resulting from immigration played a powerful role in cultivating the conditions in which women experienced abuse and social detachment. These were clearly illustrated by Domenga, a fifty-one-year-old woman from Jalisco, Mexico. She moved to the United States at the age of twenty to join her family, who had moved seven years prior. Domenga encountered an uncertain crossing through Tijuana and described an uncomfortable and expensive trip. She traveled with her younger sister, and their father picked them up in Los Angeles and drove them to meet the family in Chicago. Not long after she settled in with her family, Domenga faced a harrowing experience. She moved into her family's apartment, which was in a building with many other undocumented immigrants. She immediately felt uncomfortable in the home—her father was so strict that he wouldn't let her leave the house, make friends, or learn about her new city. In one instance, her father cornered her in the apartment, held her down, and would not let her leave. Domenga cried for help—a cry that must have been unmistakable to others residing in the small apartment building—but no one came. One night her father slipped into her bed and raped her. She screamed and screamed, but no one came to her rescue. He hit her in the face, in the head, in the mouth, and then he kept beating her. She eventually escaped and ran to her godmother's home, and she listened to her and said she would call the police. Domenga begged her not to, because she did not have legal papers and feared she would be deported. She also feared that putting her father in jail would jeopardize her family's financial security. Three decades later,

Domenga's traumatic memory rolled off her tongue—perhaps reflecting her severe depression and symptoms of PTSD.[19] In many ways, this distress became embodied in her diabetes. She talked about this violence only with the recorder turned off.

Many women communicated fears rooted in the neighborhoods in which they lived, often linking gang- and drug-related violence with family stress and immigration stress. Yolanda's story clearly depicts the breakdown of moral codes and family networks in the life of a low-income second-generation Mexican immigrant woman. In many ways, she relayed how such experiences can persist into adulthood and manifest in chronic illness. Yolanda was a forty-year-old woman whose diabetes care at the GMC was secondary to treatment for severe mental illness. She grew up in Little Village in the 1970s, with a mother who was a heroin addict and often had drug dealers and drug-abusing boyfriends in her home. Yolanda's mother beat her repeatedly, and her mother's boyfriends abused her from the age of five. She moved to her father's home at fourteen, after nearly a decade of diverting the attention of her mother's friends from her younger sister and brother. Yolanda recalled spending hours of her childhood staring out the window and much of her adolescence and adulthood abusing alcohol and other drugs. She also linked these experiences with her severe depression, which caused extreme weight fluctuations. The symptoms of PTSD and depression revealed that her psychological suffering was severe.

Yolanda's story exemplifies how a breakdown of social protection might affect the lives of the children of immigrants who are abandoned by the close networks often characterized as protective within Mexican immigrant communities. Structural factors like the lack of affordable housing and the gendered subjugation that impedes economic opportunities for single mothers may also have played an important role in Yolanda's childhood. Some scholars have argued that the absence of multigenerational and interfamilial households can contribute to increased stress within low-income families broken up due to migration. In my analysis of women's narratives, the theme of "neighborhood violence," which captured the stress stemming from feeling unsafe or scared by violence within one's physical surroundings, was more frequently reported by women who were second-generation immigrants and who resided in neighborhoods lacking a strong Mexican social fabric of support. In some cases, stressors such as gang violence and drug abuse were reported in conjunction with related forms of severe distress, such as those described in Beatriz's stories, including random shootings and the loss of a child to crossfire.

The magnitude of the interpersonal abuse reported by the women I interviewed was an impactful finding. Their narratives of interpersonal abuse were not simply about isolated incidents; instead, narratives like Domenga's and Yolanda's illustrated how the lack of legal, social, and even familial protections was a fundamental underpinning of child sexual abuse, wife battering, emotional manipulation, and verbal insults. These experiences of abuse often remained private memories for much of the women's lives, leading them to harbor negative emotions that continued, in most cases for decades, to cause prolonged emotional distress. In many cases, such experiences occurred in their youth, during childhood or early adulthood. I argue that in some sense, such violence was linked to the desperation of poverty: the numbers reported by the women in this study (and in another study of low-income Mexican immigrant women in California) were much higher than those reported by women of a different socioeconomic status.[20] It is crucial to identify such intra-ethnic differences because they demonstrate that the high rates of interpersonal abuse stem from structural and social factors, such as poverty and immigration stress, rather than from Mexican or Mexican American culture and ethnicity. Although there certainly are cultural factors that contribute to the manner in which individuals cope with and manage stress, the distribution of such social distress at the population level must be understood as a consequence of structural inequalities. Thus, interpersonal abuse, which is often gender based, may be understood to be one manifestation of such inequalities.

Yet, women's narratives from Chicago mirror multiple ethnographic studies of poor Mexican and immigrant Mexican women in the United States who face repeated experiences of abuse in their everyday lives. Specifically, domestic violence has been well documented in the Mexican context and largely framed around constructions of gender and power in Mexican marriages and associated with alcohol abuse among men.[21] Kaja Finkler's (1994) research on married Mexican women describes domestic violence, including both physical and sexual abuse, as a problem not only of gender but also of class. Finkler (1994, 33) comments: "The suffering and afflictions of women living in miserable poverty are as much connected with economic scarcity as they are with inimical social relationships with mates, family, and neighbors." Jennifer Hirsch (2003) similarly found domestic violence to be a problem for married women in Mexico and argued that the balance of gender and power within Mexican couples was shifting with modernity and migration to the United States. Both Matthew Gutmann (1999) and Seth Holmes (2013) further demonstrate the impact of immigration-linked distress with alcoholism and acting out among men. Interestingly, evidence in the United States suggests that Mexican immigrant populations report higher rates of abuse compared to the general population in the United States as well as in Mexico, and that the incidence of abuse is higher the longer the immigrants reside in the United States.[22]

In her book on gender, family, and illegality among transnational Mexicans, Deborah Boehm (2012, 89) argues that "masculinity is both reasserted and compromised because of migration between Mexico and the United States, and this, in turn, simultaneously frees and constrains women." Some women reported that they migrated to the United States to escape poverty or domestic violence and found the United States to provide a safe haven from insecurity at home. Others found similarly or more challenging experiences in their new homes but did not regret their decisions to leave. In part, the domestic violence women described throughout their stories reflects a form of symbolic violence encompassed by what Bourdieu and Wacquant (2004, 273) describe as the "domination of the dominant by his domination." In the case of the patriarchal advantage of men, this means that men are dominated by cultural and social expectations of masculinity and subconsciously try to live up to the ideals of what it means to be a man. For example, the failure to uphold cultural ideals about masculinity publicly (as a wage earner) has been associated with an increase in male aggression in the private sphere. In this sense, the social construction of what it means to be a man (and, specifically, a Mexican man in Chicago) may contribute to coping mechanisms and compensating behaviors like alcoholism, drug abuse, or domestic abuse, as men struggle to fit into an expected familial role as Mexican patriarchs that is unrealistic in the contemporary political-economic context. Such unbalanced structures force us to move beyond feminist notions of men as independent perpetrators of violence against women and to examine instead how individuals negotiate their roles of dominator and dominated within the larger political-economic and social system.

Isolation, Fear, and Health

The links between abuse, violence, and immigration were central to Mari's mental and physical suffering. Mari was a forty-year-old woman from Zacatecas who immigrated alone to the United States when she was sixteen. She was a labor migrant, moving to the United States to find work. However, when Mari encountered the border she found that the coyotes, the men who would ensure safe passage across the border for a high cost, wanted more money than she had saved for the journey. She paid for the journey through sex work—exchanging her body for her safe passage. Mari thought her dues were paid, but on arrival the coyote made her pay off her debt with him for many months before she was free to go. A thirty-five-year-old acquaintance offered to bring her to Chicago and she agreed, wanting to escape the situation in California. When she arrived in Chicago, however, Mari found a similarly tough situation. She had no friends, no family, no job. The man who accompanied her across the country informed his family that she was his girlfriend. She was alone and scared, so she accepted it and stayed with him for five years. Mari described her devastating situation: he was incredibly jealous and locked her in her room. She could not meet friends, get a job, or have any autonomy. Mari said that at one point she tried to escape but he took her shoes, her clothes, and locked her inside her bedroom. She cried and screamed, but no one came to her rescue. She responded by sleeping all the time, crying when she was awake, and eating to feel better. Mari's weight skyrocketed, and her small frame ultimately hosted 305 pounds. Eventually she convinced him to unlock the door. Their relationship improved, and he bought her food, clothes, and other necessities. Only years later did she realize that his actions were abuse. Eventually she began caregiving for acquaintances and earning money. She made friends and felt better about herself. However, she was very heavy by that point—in one year alone she had gained forty pounds. She stayed with her partner for years and left him only when he moved back to Mexico. She described feeling free after he left, although she struggled to figure out how to take the bus, speak English, and survive on her own. Five years later, Mari was thriving on her own; she still carries those compounded traumatic years, however, in her depression, anxiety, and diabetes.

Stories like Mari's are extreme, but the fear that seethes through her story is not uncommon. In many cases, fear becomes an undercurrent in women's lives that cannot be dissociated from their health, which often worsens the longer the women reside in the United States. Janet Page-Reeves and colleagues (2013) note the fundamental role of fear in structural violence that is so often overlooked in immigrant health. This fear is one way in which immigration becomes a fault line for diabetes, spurring hypervigilance and internalized distress that so often goes hidden from view and not only gets buried within the body but also disappears from epidemiological analyses of poor health.

Understanding fear as a risk factor for syndemic diabetes recognizes that we need to rethink how socially driven experiences often categorized as "culture" or "acculturation" influence the so-called Latino health paradox. This paradox is based on the surprising finding that immigrants' health deteriorates the longer they live in the United States, despite the fact that they have moved from a lower-income to a higher-income country (and based on the assumption that more wealth should produce more health). Recognizing how fear may play a role in the Latino health paradox reinforces an anthropological critique of acculturation—a concept rooted in behavioral psychology that supposes immigrant beliefs and behaviors change as they adapt to a new cultural setting. Anthropologists have argued that the acculturation construct has the potential of imposing ethnic stereotypes about what people believe and how they act;[23] by contrast, they suggest that things like fear and systemic inequality both produce heterogeneous immigrant experiences and directly fuel poor health.[24] For instance, at its most basic level, the decision to migrate from Mexico to the United States expresses an extreme marginalization within the global economy. Immigrants face structural conditions that create their undocumented status and produce violence, subjugation, and exploitation both during the migration itself and in the months and years after settling in the new country. The experience of Beatriz, a second-generation immigrant, reflects how fear penetrates immigrant's lives even when they achieve a relative economic success. It was the loss of her sons—one who lost his physical mobility and one who lost his life—from the barrel of a gun that imposed extraordinary stress on her mind and body. This stress not only drove her to "madness" (which brought to her hospitalization and the medicalization of her grief) but also created a scenario for extreme weight gain and, eventually, diabetes.

The intimate and somewhat nostalgic longing for family members—mostly sisters or mothers—in Mexico exemplifies this aspect of "acculturation" that is difficult to capture in a health survey. Many of the Mexican-born women reported longing for their families in Mexico and feeling lonely and misunderstood by their children with whom they lived in the United States. The importance of understanding the impact of these troubling feelings on health is underscored by Lisa Berkman with Ichiro Kawachi (2000) as well as with Leonard Syme (1979) and others who have taken seriously the relationship between health and feelings of social isolation. In my study, whereas some women came out and simply stated, "I'm lonely," most women described this sentiment by sharing a longing for another time or place. This narrative theme was clearly a byproduct of their migratory experiences: women spoke of longing not for Mexican food or culture, but rather for the companionship of close friends and family who understood them and their needs. At the same time, they felt that their family in the United States, often children and grandchildren, did not understand them. These feelings of loneliness and isolation were often coupled with memories of sexual abuse, and they might have been associated with the women's need to keep a difficult memory or secret from others.

Family, Caregiving, and Diabetes

Gender and power underlie many of women's narratives in this book, and they play fundamental roles in how women perceive and experience chronic illness. They were clearly at play in the experiences of abuse or subjugation that were central to many women's stories, but they also materialized in more subtle ways, such as through women's roles as caregivers, mothers, sisters, and workers. Women throughout this study prioritized their families over their selves, neglecting diabetes care in the name of family care. This was true not only in the everyday practice of caregiving but also in the allocation of finances, where women put the needs of their children, grandchildren, and spouses before their own. This also involved women's withholding their negative emotions from their children, bury-ing sadness or troubled memories from those they loved. These negative emotions were often overshadowed by worry about diabetes, and in many cases distress was linked to these past experiences rather than to chronic illness.

Women's sacrifice is a common trope in anthropology, underscoring women's roles and dedication to caregiving in the family. Gendered family dynamics situate women at the center of the home, as nurturer, caregiver, and food preparer—all tasks that have been considered "women's work" in patriarchal societies on both sides of the US–Mexico border.[25] These roles play out in the lives of women who care for their siblings during their childhoods, for their husbands in their teens, and for their own children and grandchildren for decades thereafter. For instance, in María's story, which opened chapter 1, a sixty-year-old grandmother from Vera Cruz moved to Chicago to assist her daughter in caring for her grandson. She lived with her daughter and her family, serving as caretaker of her grand-son for many years and eventually—when the tension between her daugh-ter and son-in-law reached a pinnacle—moving out of their home with her grandson. Fearing for his safety, María removed her grandson from her daughter's home and cared for his emotional, social, and economic needs. For the first time, María lived on her own and got a job as a nanny in a wealthy suburb to support her grandson. This story demonstrates how the caregiver role fueled her identity as protector and empowered her in new ways after many years of service to others. Thus, although caregiving may be perceived as a form of subjugation, it may also create opportunities for empowerment and transformation.

Many other women described their children and spouses as major stressors in their lives. Thirty percent had five or more children, and often women lived with and were dependent on their children financially. A small percentage of them lived with children, parents, or siblings who were dependent on them. In some cases, women were currently providing care for their adolescent or adult children—for example, if a child was a minor or had mental or physical disabilities. In other cases, my inter-locutors, like Beatriz, worried about their children's, or in some cases hus-band's, involvement with gangs or drugs on the streets of Chicago. Another woman described her daughter as "literally hazardous to my health."

Although women's social roles may indeed be changing as a consequence of immigration, it is clear that many women feel that their role as family caregivers is central to their identity and everyday life. Some women talked about caregiving for their grown children as well as grandchildren, often residing in a basement apartment while one or more of their children occupied the floors above. This intergenerational family arrangement provided some stability and support for women who were also navigating chronic illness. At the same time, there is a tension between the social expectation that women should care for their families and diabetes, which requires women to change their diets, increase physical activity, monitor blood glucose, and take medicines regularly.[26] Many women explained that because they commonly prepared food for and ate with family members without diabetes, modifying their diets would require their immediate family to do so. This statement put the responsibility of their own diabetes self-care in the hands of family members, and therefore reduced or excused blame for poor diabetes management; however, it also demonstrated to what extent women's decisions about their own lives are embedded within the family.

Alejandra's story illustrates this point. Unlike many women who said that diabetes was one of many issues in their lives, Alejandra found diabetes to be the most devastating. She was diagnosed with diabetes after she had a blood transfusion (which she identified as making her blood "bad"). After a decade with diabetes, she experienced worsening complications: poor eyesight, a stiff back, and tingly legs and feet that were painful to walk on. She was exhausted after walking short distances. Alejandra tried to eat fruits and vegetables, but sometimes she allowed herself french fries, or a Big Mac, or a chorizo "here and there." Determining what to eat, however, was not only a matter of desire; cost played a major role. Alejandra's husband lost his job a year before her interview with me, so purchasing food for a diabetes diet was a drain on their finances (as brown bread is more costly than white bread). Her dedication to caring for diabetes, however, changed once her daughter was diagnosed. Alejandra worried that her daughter would suffer in ways that she had suffered, and this caused her to change the family diet and care for her daughter in ways she had never cared for herself. Alejandra's story is not uncommon, and in many cases women discussed how they had lovingly cared for husbands, parents, and siblings with diabetes differently than they had for themselves.

Finally, women repeatedly described social trauma as more stressful than diabetes. This is an important point, because the biomedical literature so often links distress among people with chronic illness to the medical condition as opposed to addressing social suffering or a combination of social and medical problems. For instance, when I approached Gloria in the GMC to ask her to participate in an interview about stress and diabetes, her son's girlfriend, who was accompanying her to the clinic, said, "Oh yes, she could definitely benefit from speaking to someone about her diabetes." What I observed, however, was that, although she said she could "not accept that I have diabetes because it is so grave," her distress was more complex, involving a story threaded with child abuse, migration to escape it, and a new life in Chicago. Many years later, Gloria stated that the anger she felt when she remembered the past was too powerful. Flashbacks associated with a car accident also persisted into the present. She had not visited a medical center for many years, and it was the physician in the emergency room who received her after the car crash who diagnosed her diabetes. She explained that her fear, nerves, and emotions caused her diabetes (specifically discussing *susto*, a rattling fright resulting from the crash). Perhaps because of her depression, Gloria said she spent most of her time alone, largely isolating herself from family and friends. It was very clear that her family was worried about her, but she complained that no one understood her pain. This might reflect the fact that her children did not know about her emotionally difficult past—but she never spoke about it. Whereas her emotions and chronic illness were visible, their deep-seated causes were buried from sight, and so it was easier for her family members to interpret her suffering as located in the present.

Rethinking Diabetes in Chicago

Rethinking diabetes in the United States requires that we consider how the social world is deeply embedded in medical conditions like diabetes. The VIDDA syndemic offers a narratively centered interpretation of how social and psychological suffering are embedded in diabetes experiences among low-income Mexican immigrant women in Chicago. Social traumas linked to immigration, gender subjugation, and poverty cannot be dissociated from diabetes among these women, because they were so salient to their everyday lives. Creating space within the clinical sphere—with a nurse, a social worker, or perhaps a new cadre of counselors at the primary care level—can offer an opportunity for women to *speak through diabetes* and share how their social, individual, and emotional worlds may affect their sickness and health. Thus, diabetes is not only a measure of insulin resistance; it is a social experience and the embodiment of a stressful life.

Understanding VIDDA provides an opportunity to think about how syndemic diabetes may manifest across contexts. Returning to the VIDDA syndemic visual from figure 3, the complex biosocial framework that shapes syndemics serves to orient my analysis of syndemic suffering in the following chapters. Structural factors shape the ways in which people can move securely in the world, and they include issues ranging from unemployment to laws around immigration to unsafe neighborhoods. Sociocultural factors shape how people live in the world through the prism of gender inequality, racism, and social networks. Conflict and support both shape relationship factors, which can further influence how people negotiate structural racism and sociocultural challenges. Finally, individual factors are also fundamental in VIDDA, as foods, feelings, friends, and social roles fundamentally transform how people experience and interact in the world. Yet, how these factors manifest within diverse contexts requires an analytic scrutiny of what syndemic interactions become relevant among people facing different challenges along lines of gender, class, and race.

3

DELHI

Meena

Meena opened the door to her flat in a pink *salwar kameez* and big looped gold earrings. Her eyes were encircled by wrinkles and her dry skin was framed by carefully oiled black hair tied back in plaits. She lived in a modest two-bedroom flat in northern Delhi. This home was nicer than the one she had lived in before they received the government-subsidized flat. Meena and her husband shared their home with two sons, two daughters, a daughter-in-law, and their children. This joint family arrangement was common among the low-income families like Meena's that we interviewed. Even though the apartment was crowded, it was much sturdier and secure than the slum from which they had moved. Meena represented the one in three interlocutors in Delhi who resided in government housing—the rest lived in wealthier enclaves. Meena invited us into her home because she routinely met there the research team for another study she had engaged in for more than a year. She warmly welcomed Sneha,

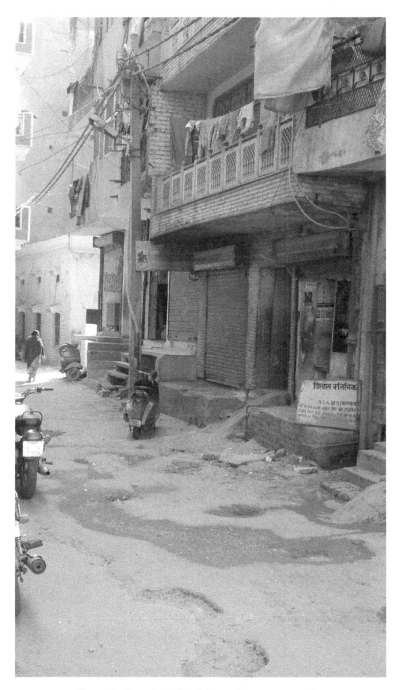

Figure 4. Street in Old Delhi resettlement community.
Photo by Allam Ashraf.

my research assistant. They sat huddled together on a cot on her cement veranda overlooking Old Delhi, speaking quietly in Hindi. Nobody else was home.

Meena was born and had enjoyed a calm childhood in a village in Haryana, only a short bus ride from Delhi. She first came to Delhi to marry at the age of twelve. Entering her husband's home introduced a radical shift in her life. She expounded on her fear of her mother-in-law, who routinely abused her emotionally and verbally. She also withheld food for "up to two days" and routinely pushed her out of the home. This abuse fostered conflict with her new husband, although Meena describes quietly accepting the abuse. This is not uncommon in Delhi, where many women follow tradition by moving in with their husbands' families after marriage to rear their children with intergenerational support. Yet, becoming mothers at such a young age can have profound consequences for young women who hold minimal power in the household. For years, Meena sought refuge for long periods with her parents. She stated that her mother-in-law "spoiled my whole married life."

The friction with her mother-in-law was not only emotional but also financial. Her husband had a good job, as he worked in the postal department for the government. Her mother-in-law perceived their independence as a threat, however, and collected his paycheck to prevent the couple from becoming autonomous. She said that her husband's mother feared "all of my husband's money would come to me" and therefore "always tried to create friction between me and my husband." Meena remembers this time with deep sorrow, explaining that "she was successful in her intentions. My husband did not like me at all . . . [because I was] a villager and I was not beautiful." Meena cried softly throughout the interview.

Over time, however, Meena's situation changed. Her husband's younger brother was married and another woman entered their joint family home, shifting the power dynamic. Meena explained that her parents assured her for years that "one day things will be fine and I should have patience." Indeed, "the day came when my younger sister-in-law came" and "she started replying back to my mother-in-law and did not listen to her. Then she realized in comparison that I was good." Things also improved when her mother-in-law was diagnosed with cancer. Meena explained that after the diagnosis, her mother-in-law fell sick, and she and her husband took care of her. Through this difficult transition, her mother-in-law "realized that she did bad to me and started to bless me in the last moments of her life." Following her mother-in-law's transformation, her husband also "apologized to me that he did wrong to me."

Then, however, Meena paused and asked, "What will I do with the apology?" She went on to explain that despite some brief periods of relative calm, her relationship with her husband did not improve: "I am stressed because my husband turned to alcohol after his mother's death. He abuses me and shouts at me when he is drunk. He has stopped hitting me like he used to do." His alcoholism did not only affect her physically, but it also caused her family to "lose so much property" and to experience financial insecurity—as she explained, "We do not have any savings." This financial insecurity has produced a prolonged stress in Meena's life and caused her preoccupation with finding a new home. At the time of the interview, Meena was living in government housing associated with her husband's employment. Because he was soon to retire, before long they would be forced to find a new home, which was costly and daunting to her. Other financial problems also plagued Meena and her family, such as her brother's outstanding debt.

Meena also described many moments of love, strength, and pride associated with motherhood and caregiving. When asked who she was closest to among her sons and daughters, Meena exclaimed, "I am closest to goddess Durga—mother of a lion!" She said she maintained a close relationship with her eldest son, who resided with her with his wife and two children. She worried constantly about her daughters—not only about their happiness but also about their safety as married women. She grieved that their mothers-in-law treated them poorly, and she felt "sad for them." Meena noted that she maintained a strong relationship with her daughter-in-law who resided with her.

Meena discovered her diabetes during an intense period of her life. She was very close to both daughters, but especially the youngest. The eldest was married at an early age; the youngest lived with her for many years, and they frequently went shopping together. Meena looked at the floor when she said that her youngest daughter "used to love me a lot and she was very funny." Just before her youngest daughter's marriage, Meena "fell sick." She became "sleep deprived" and "very nervous" and felt her "palpitations increased." When she "started to sweat and feel dizzy," Meena's son brought her to a private doctor.

The doctor diagnosed her with high cholesterol, high blood pressure, and high blood sugar. Meena quickly responded to treatment and took medication for hypertension for one year. But her diabetes diagnosis frightened her. She "cried a lot" and asked, "What kind of disease is this?" She meditated on the thought that "now I have to limit my eating." This change was perhaps the hardest for Meena. Reflecting back, however, Meena stated how diabetes was "so normal now." She no longer took medication but routinely met her doctor for checkups. Her eldest son paid 50 Rupees per visit out-of-pocket. Without this financial support, she would have had to seek diabetes care exclusively at a government clinic, which she detested because of the "long queues." Patients wait many hours to see their physicians at the large public hospitals as well as in smaller clinics. During the two years of managing her diabetes, Meena took medications for only "three months," despite the fact that her glucose remains high. She felt fatalistic, commenting: "Even if I go now for a checkup, it will come [back] high." Meena stated that her doctor said her diabetes was "normal" and her elder daughter said "there is nothing to worry about" and diabetes "is normal these days."

Meena continued to meditate on how she would change her diet. "To eat normal foods" she said, "I don't eat much, don't take sugar. I left tea. It's been two years since I had tea." She stopped eating starches, including rice and potato, and she said "my daughter-in-law doesn't let me eat anything that can raise my sugar level." In terms of social support, she described how her daughter-in-law "cooks separately for me" and "if sometime I feel like having something fried like *aloo tikki,* then she cooks with soybean and spinach. She is very smart. She makes food for me like that only, with soya, chopped spinach, tamarind paste, and curd every two or three Sundays." She also depended on her daughter-in-law to seek routine medical care. When asked if her husband ever helped with her diabetes care, Meena responded, "No, he doesn't even care."

The interview closed with Meena explaining that diabetes had become common among her neighbors. She walked Sneha to the door, and Sneha thanked her warmly. Meena beamed as Sneha left her home. She said she felt lighter and unburdened after spending time speaking about her experiences. I met Sneha not far from Meena's small government flat.

We walked through the narrow street sandwiched between government housing on each side. Families sat in bright-colored doorways watching the afternoon pass.

Methods and Context

Meena's and the others' narratives were collected in Delhi, one of India's famous megacities with nearly 18 million people inhabiting the larger urban area. Delhi has been continuously inhabited by people since the sixth century BC, and the legacy of human occupation is visible in the city's archeological sites amid beautiful gardens, modern buildings, and buttressing slums. As the parliamentary seat, South Delhi features planned gardens and elite neighborhoods, whereas Old Delhi (to the north, where Meena resides) maintains more densely populated neighborhoods with visibly fewer trees and many more families struggling to make ends meet. Delhi is both a reflection of modern India and microcosm in its own right. It is sprawling and dense, putrid and sweet, colorful and dank. Its inequality is visible and vast.[1]

Like many global cities, Delhi is extraordinarily heterogeneous in terms of class, ethnicity, and religion. Delhi, along with India more broadly, has been continuously resettled and remade through centuries of colonialism, from the Mughal Empire to the British Raj. Each time a new colonial power took hold, a reconstitution of the city ensued. When India won its independence from the British, the Partition of 1947 spurred a mass migration, with Muslims moving en masse from Delhi to Pakistan and Hindus flooding the city. Today, four of every five residents are Hindu, with smaller communities of Sikhs, Muslims, Jains, Christians, and others. Finding longstanding family legacies in the city is less common; it is a city of immigrants. This too contributes to the fluidity and heterogeneity of the urban space.

Meena is one of sixty men and women residing in Old Delhi whom my team interviewed, and many of them moved to Delhi during childhood or early adulthood. I spent a year in Delhi, working closely with colleagues at the Public Health Foundation of India (PHFI) as a research fellow funded by the National Institutes of Health Fogarty International Center. I was selected to work at PHFI with the Center for Cardio-Metabolic Risk

Reduction in South Asia (CARRS) Surveillance Study, which had recently formed a National Heart, Lung, and Blood Institute (NHLBI) Center of Excellence (COE)[2] to combat chronic diseases. Mine was an unusual role for an anthropologist, but the team of epidemiologists and clinicians were intrigued to have a social scientist investigate why diabetes was materializing among low-income groups and how their experiences might be different from those of elite or middle-income urban Indians.

At the time, India was known as the diabetes capital of the world. The large number of people living with diabetes in India, compared to many nations with relatively higher diabetes prevalence, is in part a reflection of the country's large population: one in every seven humans resides in South Asia. The rapid escalation of diabetes in India, however, reflects swift social, cultural, and economic transformations that have swept through the region. The escalation of diabetes initially hugged the cities, although rural diabetes incidence and prevalence has also increased in past decades. As people migrated from rural communities to urban areas, globalization's grip on postcolonial India changed how people interacted, thought, ate, and moved. With a growing middle class and the opening of international markets, the types of food people desired and cooked and the way people moved in the world—on their way to work, in the home, among others—transformed everyday life. These changes affected not only the elites but also lower-income Indians. How the forces of modernization might materialize in the everyday lives of urban Indians and how income might influence such experiences were for me crucial research questions pointed at understanding how diabetes becomes syndemic.

Working from the CARRS Cohort Study, my colleague Roopa Shivashankar and I identified a number of people with diabetes residing in three adjacent neighborhoods in Old Delhi. We decided to control the study somewhat by only interviewing people who self-identified as Hindus, the largest religious group in Delhi. We invited twenty to twenty-five people from each neighborhood to participate. One neighborhood was affluent, showcasing its stature by a large gate and a number of private homes for its residents. Another neighborhood was middle class, and it hosted wealthier families who lived in single-family homes or apartments; these homes were more modest than the gilded gated communities but much larger than government housing. The last neighborhood was a collection of government-sponsored homes for people who relocated in

Delhi from the slums, known as a resettlement community; many of these homes had only a sleeping room and a kitchen, some had two floors, and others had open space on the roof.

We called one hundred eligible people enrolled in the CARRS parent study and residing in one of the three neighborhoods to schedule a visit. Sixty people invited us to their homes, and few eligible study participants declined to participate. I trained two research assistants to conduct the interviews over a period of two weeks; these two researchers—Sneha Sharma and Allam Ashraf—were gender matched (an important convention within Hindu contexts) to prevent any uncomfortable feelings during the discussion of sensitive issues, including emotions or memories of social traumas. I accompanied Sneha and Ashraf on the first several interviews, but we soon realized that it was more productive for them to visit the study participants without me because our interlocutors were timid to speak in my presence and seemed to open up when I stepped out. I maintained an ongoing dialogue with them about the interviews and closely reviewed their daily field notes; these notes were one- to two-page reflections on various aspects of the interview, and they enabled me to remain closely engaged.

A CARRS team member accompanied Sneha and Ashraf to facilitate the first contact with each interlocutor. Sneha and Ashraf introduced themselves, described the study as focused on stress and diabetes, and scheduled an interview for a later date.[3] In some cases, if the interlocutor was available, the interview was conducted the same day. Our interlocutors engaged with Sneha or Ashraf for one to two hours. In some cases, Sneha felt more comfortable with Ashraf accompanying her to the interview; in these cases, Ashraf sat outside or in another room to provide privacy. These two hours comprised the life history narrative interviews, followed by the administration of the Hopkins Symptoms Checklist.[4]

Meena and others described myriad challenges they confronted in their daily lives, outlining the cascading effects of family problems, financial problems, and social challenges that were not disconnected from their diabetes or other medical problems. Meena's narrative, however, represents primarily the experience of low-income individuals and can be sharply juxtaposed to the experience of people who were wealthier, residing in middle-income and high-income neighborhoods. Nearly everyone in the study had been married at some point in their lives, was Hindu, and was forty years of age or older. People like Meena who resided in the resettlement community completed less education and maintained lower incomes than those from wealthier neighborhoods. This group also reported more depression (55 percent) compared to those from middle-income (38 percent) and high income (29 percent) neighborhoods. More than half of those interviewed, unlike Meena, had been diagnosed with diabetes ten or more years before the interview; more than two-thirds of the wealthier participants had known they had diabetes for a decade.

Our interlocutors described between two and five different types of stressful experiences throughout their lives, with the average of three and many overlapping experiences (see figure 5 for the lowest-income women only). The challenges people described, however, differed by both gender and income in important ways: The wealthiest group indicated that most distress was spun from financial problems, personal health, loss of a family member, family conflict, and concern for their children's futures. The middle-income group described concern for their children's futures, family conflict, personal health, financial conflict, joint family problems, and work-related concerns to be the most pressing stresses in their lives. The lowest-income group reported stress over their children's futures, family conflict, family health, children's potential for marriage, personal health, and financial futures to be the most stressful issues in their lives.[5] In summary, social stressors associated with meeting expectations regarding children's futures, financial security, and family were the most common across income groups, but how these subjective stresses were realized in people's lives varied in important ways.

The differences among these groups provide important insights into how and why the lowest-income group may differently experience diabetes, distress, and social factors amid chronic illness. For instance, concern for one's children's future as well as family stress and financial insecurities were described by nearly all of our interlocutors, regardless of income or gender; however, how people fretted about these things manifested in notably different ways. The wealthier interlocutors described achieving economic and social success through buying goods, arranging marriages that might bring upward mobility, and dissolving the joint household. Lower-income interlocutors, in contrast, described the stress of meeting the social expectation of paying for a home, of saving enough money to pay dowry and arrange a good marriage for their children, and of supporting their children's needs,

Life stressors in Delhi (low-income women only)

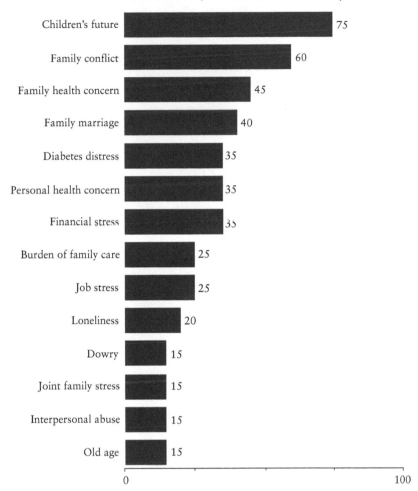

Figure 5. Life stressors in Delhi (low-income women only)

such as paying for school. Low-income women in particular described the repercussions of interpersonal abuse and alcoholism, whereas wealthier women described a deep-seated loneliness linked with the dissolution of joint family living arrangements. Similarly, whereas one-quarter of our interlocutors reported diabetes distress, only those from the low-income community reported co-occurring depression, and these respondents also described complications with diabetes. These individuals were also more likely to have delayed seeking care due to cost. Through this analysis, an economic argument around the poverty-diabetes nexus that cultivates syndemics emerged, incorporating the impacts of globalization, ideas about social progress, and the challenges to get by in the global city.

Syndemic Suffering in Delhi

Syndemic suffering in Delhi mirrored syndemic suffering in Chicago in meaningful ways. Perhaps the closest alignment with VIDDA was among the low-income women who described how the chronicities of poverty shaped their life chances, social traumas, and gendered subjugation in the family. These individual-level factors can be situated within macro-social forces—much like in VIDDA—that structured opportunities for men and women, expectations about success and opportunities for their children, and financial stress. Yet, important factors along the macro-micro nexus seemingly transformed how syndemic suffering was experienced and embodied in Delhi compared to Chicago. The most obvious force was the ways in which culture change influenced how people perceived and worked toward their families' social and economic progress. This distinctly shaped experiences with stress, food, caregiving, and diabetes, and their interpretations. The narratives also provided a window into how diabetes is both gendered and experienced across income groups, revealing a fundamentally different experience among those who face syndemic poverty, diabetes, and distress.

For Meena, these complexities came together throughout her life course in meaningful ways. Meena's most stressful memory was tied to an arranged marriage in her youth. Leaving her childhood home, which she described as a somewhat reflective and quiet period, was juxtaposed to a joint family environment steeped in tension and power imbalances between Meena and her husband as well as her mother-in-law. The gendered subjectivities within the home were related not only to marital expectations but also to her role in the family associated with her age. Her experience was transformed as the power dynamic shifted when, first, a younger woman entered the family, and second, her mother-in-law's position of power was threatened by terminal illness. This was a point of transformation for Meena within the family, when her vulnerable position shifted and she gained more authority. However, her husband's physical abuse was stymied only momentarily, and his despair in response to losing his mother threatened their financial security. Meena discovered that the destabilization of her family dynamic due to her youngest child's marriage— for her, another loss of status as mother within the home—was more stress than she was able to bear. This anxiety inspired a hospital visit, whereby following a number of medical tests she found she had many of the characteristics of cardio-metabolic problems. With this new biomedical reality, Meena appeared to accept her diagnosis of diabetes and to harness the power of family support by way of her daughter-in-law's advocating for her, recognizing diabetes as something that is "normal these days."

The following analysis of syndemic suffering shows how not only culture but also gender and income shifted how people perceived and experienced diabetes in Delhi. First, there was an inherent cultural difference in how people spoke about diabetes in Delhi compared to Chicago, with many people normalizing diabetes in their everyday speech. Second, culture change linked to the globalization of ideas and everyday practices materialized differently across interlocutors with divergent incomes, from the enactment of cultural rituals—such as dowry—to expectations about what it meant to live a good life. Third, poverty and structural violence in Delhi produce a distinct form of syndemic suffering that aligns diabetes with VIDDA. Meena and other low-income women often described social traumas in their lives parallel to those shared by women in Chicago, such as violence, isolation, and abuse. Finally, family dynamics were interrelated with diabetes, creating a unique role in how people perceived, prioritized, and cared for their diabetes. This was found across all narratives, although it manifested differently depending on the availability of extra income. The rest of this chapter draws from multiple interlocutors' stories to consider how syndemic suffering in Delhi is distinctly local, while at the same time illuminating some global trends.

Culture, Modernity, and Diabetes

I have argued that one way in which syndemic suffering matters is in how diabetes becomes a social experience after diagnosis. This manifested in a distinctly cultural way in Delhi, where—as opposed to sharing the shame and stigma so common in the West[6]—most interlocutors reaffirmed how diabetes was "normal" and "not a disease," noting that "everyone has diabetes," that it can "happen to anyone," and that "this is just the way the world is." Many emphasized the inevitable nature of diabetes, for example by saying, "It's a disease, anything can happen, anyone can suffer" and "it was my fate." Others stated that at the time of their diabetes diagnosis, their friends and family members comforted them by emphasizing that the disease was very common: "Most of the people have diabetes, in every house." By recognizing diabetes as part of the social fabric of modern life, people may diminish the self-blame associated with the condition and identify instead a broader social culprit.

This social culprit may indeed be social change. For instance, Ravi, a middle-income man, described how the global turn influenced how he perceived success and social status. Ravi began his description by speaking about what caused him "tension" (also described as *tenśan,* or *tenshun*)—a local idiom of distress. He talked about "the status factor": "We need to have a car, a bungalow, so much money to survive. I guess people are running fast to have money and the reason is if you don't have all of these things, then you would not be respected in society. If you don't have status, you will not be able to arrange a good marriage." In his construction of what defines a good life, social status was linked to material goods, but nearly every time these material goods led back to the need to find a good spouse for one's children. Ravi went on to describe how social status was imperative to match with a good family: "I would also get my daughter married some day and I would definitely look for a guy who has a good house, a good job, family background. So many people now have a compulsion to maintain a status factor."

India has so often been a test case for theories of the sociocultural impact of rapid economic change. Arjun Appadurai's iconic *Modernity at Large* (1996) uses India as a microcosm of the global cultural flows that reveal how interconnected humans have become through finances, ideas, people, goods, and technologies that are in constant motion. This perspective works against the idea of India as one static entity and instead suggests how global ideas transform individual lives as well as families and prevailing cultural beliefs. In other words, this framework challenges the notion that modernity transpires in the same way in every nation, every province within that nation, or every family—despite its global authority. The varied ways in which people in Delhi perceived such global flows to materialize in their everyday lives were central to how people engaged with these political-economic and cultural shifts. For instance, in contrast to Ravi, many-lower income interlocutors grieved their inability to meet the cultural expectations about dowry to pay for a good match for their children. Families worried not only about attracting a good marriage, but also about having substantial financial resources to pay for a marriage at all. This tension revealed a complex balance of old and new ways of being, of "traditional" and "modern" expectations for being a good mother, father, daughter, or son. This divergence also pointed to a cultural dissonance in how social and economic changes were experienced and interpreted along economic lines, with the lowest-income families being nearly crippled by the financial obligation of dowry within a global society of increasing material prioritization.

These broad cultural changes are inextricably linked to the policies of economic liberalization initiated in India since the 1980s and early 1990s, which have spurred cultural shifts in consumption practices and economic gains that have turned the lower-income population into the new middle class.[7] The notion of expanding commodities as a badge of honor is one example of how culture change has manifested among middle-income, and in some cases lower-income, urban Indians. This was described by many middle- and upper-class interlocutors like Ravi, who described how their children would become "independent" and have a "good life" only if a better income could afford them the materialities of success in a global society. Such cultural shifts also manifest in the fact that young people hold different values and beliefs about what defines a successful life than their parents.[8] Many of our interlocutors pointed to the fact that the fast-paced uptake of social change among young people fostered intergenerational conflict as young people more quickly adapted to global ideas and opportunities.

Moreover, many people connected culture change with diabetes. Rajeev, who resided in the middle-income neighborhood, described the intricate link between diabetes and these global shifts. Rajeev contrasted a previous life in which "people worked so hard" that diabetes "was so uncommon" to the social reality of the present day. He mused how people once did things by hand and now would use automated machines. They used to walk and now they drove. They once used hand pumps and wells for water and now they used taps. Rajeev said, "This modern, high-tech era has had some bad effects on our health." Rajeev also made an important point that was linked not only to the physical world but also to the impact of social and psychological experiences on the human body. He brought up the important concept of tension, which is a common idiom of distress that often incorporates depressive symptoms and communicates social discord in its very definition. Rajeev described how, looking back two or three decades, people did not experience tension, which he connected explicitly with living in the modern era. They did not experience diabetes. He said, "I guess the automated advanced age is the biggest source of any kind of diseases."

Gender, Family, and Tension

Pooja was encouraged by her teachers to complete her schooling, but she had to drop out when her grandfather and uncle were murdered for "political reasons" and her father shouldered the burden of leading the family. He quickly married Pooja off. By the age of nineteen Pooja had her first child, resided with her husband's family, and was deeply involved in her new domestic life. Her eldest was seven by the time Sneha interviewed her, and she described the escalating financial pressure of raising two boys. What was most distressing for Pooja was the fact that her husband was unemployed and not interested in finding a job outside the home. As a result, she frequently had to depend on her mother-in-law for money to care for her two sons, and this caused an uncomfortable tension between them. This stress was linked to the gender oppression that permeated her life, which was embodied in her comment, "I never want a girl child, not because I am gender biased but because I know being a girl what problems she would have to face." She said she had never experienced interpersonal violence; she had always felt relatively safe at home during her childhood and her marriage. More than anything, she felt powerless. Her in-laws provided her with food and clothing, but she described having to repeatedly advocate for her sons so that they could get a good education. She repeated that education was as important as the food and clothing, for which her in-laws willingly paid. Pooja described feeling tension because she was sad about her family situation. She also shared that she frequently spoke with her sister, who remained a close confidant, revealing a strong source of social and emotional support outside of the tense marital home.

Pooja's story exemplifies how the household, recognized broadly within anthropology as an institution of moral order and cultural reproduction,[9] serves as a vehicle of oppression for many women. Meena, like other low-income women in urban India, described the complexities of powerlessness within her household: She was overworked, lonely, enduring abuse from a husband or mother-in-law, and caring for family members struggling through illness. Veena Das and colleagues (2012, 1671) argue that the household is the "constitutive unit for understanding the link between socioeconomic characteristics [and] adverse events such as sickness and child mortality and mental health" in urban India. In this sense, the family serves as a unit to measure syndemic suffering in Delhi: Here, health and sickness are (re)produced within strict hierarchies that determine who holds the power and the purse strings to maintain health and thwart disease. Das and colleagues (2012, 1669) found that women express how "care-giving functions made them much more vulnerable to misfortunes" because they held minimal power and had to "depend on others [such as their sister or mother] to help them tide over difficult situations." In these cases, it may be impossible for women to reject the family or their role within the family, even when they suffer abuse from family members. Many women felt isolated, powerless, and unsupported in their roles as caregivers in their husband's homes. These social factors were closely knit with tension and further compromised by poverty.

Many expressed tension as a consequence of family dynamics, financial insecurities, and the stress linked to culture change and financial obligations described by Pooja, Ravi, and Meena. The role of tension in chronic illness has been the research focus of two anthropologists who have investigated how the social world becomes embodied, or "absorbed," in diabetes. Lesley Jo Weaver (2017) has argued that tension in Delhi is produced by social relationships that do not conform to cultural norms (especially those described by Pooja and others within the family), acutely stressful economic strife, and problems with culture change. Similarly, Harris Solomon (2016) has described tension as a semi-permanent form of stress that cannot be dissociated from those navigating metabolic changes from socioeconomic stress, including the difficulty of finding money to eat or purchase medicines. In these ways, tension resembles a low-grade depressive experience that is socially and psychologically embedded in the macro-micro nexus through which people navigate social stress alongside chronic illness, care-seeking, and self-care. Tension, a fundamental part of the diabetes-poverty syndemic in Delhi, is one example of how psychological suffering reflects social discord that is also closely tied to the body. Somatic symptoms are commonly linked to tension—from insomnia to racing thoughts, loss of appetite, and elevated blood pressure. This cultural idiom therefore serves as a broader social commentary on how everyday stress becomes embodied.

Pooja's story also exemplifies how many aspired to move beyond those factors that caused them tension. Pooja had a palpable yearning for schooling. Sneha described speaking at length about possible ways in which Pooja might complete her education. She was keen to finish coursework and take exams so that she might apply to college. When she spoke about her children, her primary goal was for them to attend university rather than drop out of school and continue the family business. She said the only barrier for her was the fact that she was not supposed to leave her home without her husband.

Joint family discord was often the cause of tension and in many cases depression. This finding was commonly expressed among all women, although it manifested differently depending on income. This may be exemplified best by the story of Sandana—a wealthy woman residing in a large home with, as Sneha described it, "a fancy sofa, paintings, and furniture that occupied the whole place." Despite this relative luxury, Sandana described her home as the cause of her depression. Sandana had lived in another upscale neighborhood in Delhi, where she had resided with her extended family. After an argument with her brother-in-law, however, Sandana and her husband were forced to sell their portion of the home to the brother-in-law at a low price and leave the family. She explained that she had faced other discord in her life, such as an abuse during childhood and the illness of her husband, who had battled cancer at a young age (although he had survived and they maintained a positive relationship). Social and familial dismissal, however, remained the most powerful disapproval that she could not shake. Sandana often socially isolated herself because she was so sad about losing her family and community. Yet, Sandana's children supported her immensely with her diabetes and routinely brought her to a private clinic for care. She remained worried about her weight and diet, stating that she would never reveal her actual weight. She said she had thought about walking regularly but was too busy. Offhand, she stated that she might join a gym.

Whereas Sandana revealed one wealthy woman's despair over the dissolution of a joint family, both Meena and Pooja exemplify joint family conflict within lower-income households. These tensions often centered on interpersonal relationships between mothers-in-law and daughters-in-law, and they mostly involved disputes over raising children and doing household chores. In many ways, such disputes reveal clearly changing ideals about gender, women's roles, and intergenerational dynamics.[10] One wealthy woman said she could not escape her patriarchal home because, as she stated, "All the time I was busy with housework." The fact that she was upset about consuming her life in the home revealed an evolving notion of gender and power that was stressful not only between spouses but also between generations. This finding reflects an important aspect of culture change, because in a country such as India where the family is prioritized over the individual, family discord dislocates one's social world and creates emotional distress.[11] It also reveals a critical dimension of subjective social stress within wealthier families that may continue to escalate as traditional dynamics within joint family households are challenged.

The tension over arranging marriages and funding dowries exemplifies how low-income women expressed distress differently from wealthy women. For instance, one woman described her life as largely calm; she had a positive relationship with her husband and her diabetes was under control. The only thing that caused her stress was finding good spouses for her children. Another low-income man described the major stress in his life as the fear that his daughter would be unhappy and mistreated in her marriage, stating, "I should have found her a better family." Preet, whose alcoholic husband caused all her troubles, was consumed with worry because she could not pay for rent or food, did not own a home, and wanted her daughters to finish their schooling. She was also consumed with the fact that she was too financially insecure to find her daughters a good marriage (or to pay the dowry). Thus, Preet had to balance her pride and expectation that her daughters would advance in school with a constant fretting about paying for their marriages. This cultural dissonance reveals a powerful juncture in Indian society, in which expectations of change (such as education) confront expectations of tradition (such as marriage).

Meena and others discussed how dowry-induced stress affected not only the lives of the parents but also those of their children. Arranged marriages are common among Indian families, and the duty often falls to parents such as Preet. In many ways, as Ravi's narrative reveals, many perceive a good marriage as a vehicle for elevating the social status of the family. Yet, social expectations of dowry payments have increased exponentially over the past several years, and the increased financial burden affects the purses of not only the wealthy but also the poor. Although dowry was outlawed in 1969, it continues to be widely practiced across India and remains part of the social fabric, further crippling the financial situation of many working-class families.[12] The social and emotional stress imposed by this social obligation, therefore, cannot be dissociated from other aspects of family life, including other financial needs like paying for medical bills.

Geeta, on the other hand, described how such notions might be changing. Like other low-income women, she lost sleep over concerns about saving for dowry and arranging her eldest daughter's marriage. Financially, she was worried that she might have to sell her parents' property to afford her daughter's marriage. When Sneha asked if she would relax once the marriage was finalized—as the preparations were in the final stages—she said that she would then worry about how her daughter's in-laws would treat her daughter. She insisted that marriage introduced too many problems (as she had found early in her own marriage). Yet, she provided a different viewpoint on her second daughter, who was in medical school. Geeta said that they wouldn't have to worry so much about her because women are more attractive when they have a professional life. She also stated that her son was more interested in investing in his daughter's education than in saving for dowry. These interesting points suggest a potential shift in the ways in which families prioritize women's success in lieu of hefty dowries.

Diabetes and Interactional Suffering

Geeta's story also provides one example of how caregiving—for children, parents, spouses, and siblings—consumed many women's lives, resulting in a worsening of their own health. They would provide care even when they themselves suffered from a potentially debilitating chronic illness such as diabetes, depression, or an overlap of the two. Geeta exemplified this by describing how she spent most of her time caring for her husband's brother and mother-in-law. Geeta took her brother-in-law, recently diagnosed with cancer, to frequent appointments, and she generally supported him throughout this new life-threatening condition. Previously, she had cared for her mother-in-law, who had diabetes, for many years. This is why Geeta did not fear diabetes and commented that every family has someone with diabetes. She said that she knew not to eat sweets, and that her children cared for her diet. She dismissed her own role in self-regulating her diet, stating that if she could she would eat fried food, rice, and potatoes. Although Geeta admitted that diabetes might have had some effect on her life trajectory, she explained that she wouldn't worry because she felt well.

Geeta's story reveals what Weaver (2016, 10) describes as "trans-personal suffering," where suffering incorporates not only the complex psychological and physical problems of individuals but also the social and medical needs of their family members. This complex family dynamic was illustrated by two moments of Meena's story: first, when her position within the family was renegotiated by the terminal illness of her mother-in-law, and second, when her own diagnosis shifted her focus from her family to her illness and her daughter-in-law started to accompany her. In both cases, the intergenerational transfer of social roles and household duties had a profound impact on the tension Meena felt in her everyday life. These instances brought forms of relief for Meena. However, in many cases, transpersonal suffering may spur more caregiving responsibilities on top of more fear surrounding what might happen with one's own illness, as was the case for Geeta after she observed her mother-in-law suffer from complications. These issues are particularly salient in families with fewer means, because they would not seek outside domestic support and instead would require the labor of another family member (most likely a woman of lower rank). Within families with greater means, such social disruption may emerge less frequently due to the possibility to seek outside help, such as a paid caregiver or housekeeper.[13]

Putting family needs in front of personal needs can have a major impact on syndemic suffering. For instance, Chokkanathan (2009) has argued that interpersonal abuse may be higher than reported among women in India and closely linked to elevated depression among women when compared to men. Interpersonal abuse may affect more than depressive symptoms, too, and Claire Snell-Rood (2015) has argued that many women in Delhi slums do not eat as a response to domestic violence, marital fights and fears, and stress related to caregiving.[14] Snell-Rood's scholarship complicates the complex notion of eating and food insecurity, suggesting that women may negotiate power within the home (associated with controlling food) to gain a form of personal control amid a stressful family life. Because experiences of abuse are so widespread, the act of displacing food to respond to stress, violence, or caregiving may be a common practice. This comment returns the focus to the role of stress amid hunger and crisis, and it requires that we take seriously the role of embodied suffering in insulin resistance.

These gendered dimensions of embodied suffering were further expressed in women's narratives of interpersonal abuse. For instance, one in four women reported interpersonal abuse, compared to one in ten men. This was slightly higher among low-income women, with one in three reporting abuse. Such undisclosed abuse may play a part in the increased levels of psychological distress among women—something that is not different from what we found in Chicago, where many women had carried narratives of abuse with them for years without communicating their suffering with others. Similarly, women's narratives of abuse—physical, sexual, and verbal—are most likely underreported or normalized and swept under the rug.

Putting the family first also mediates how people care for their diabetes, something so commonly linked to self-care. Geeta's example of caring for her mother-in-law's diabetes is one way in which women prioritized the needs of other family members as an extension of their familial caregiving role. On the other hand, Geeta's description of how her children attended to her dietary needs for her diabetes exemplified how she put her prescriptions for self-care in the hands of others. The expectation that one's children will care for their parents and in-laws was woven into the narratives of caring for chronic illness. Placing the burden of care on family members may, in some ways, remove self-blame and release some of the stress of living with chronic illness. In this way, the family can provide a sort of emotional cushion for those dealing with diabetes.

There is also an important economic dimension to these points about putting family before the self that may have a major impact on diabetes. For instance, wealthier participants knew many people with diabetes and were much more likely to speak about diabetes as common or to have a family member or friend with the condition. Yet, those with lower incomes were less familiar with diabetes, had fewer family members with the condition, and were more likely to have been diagnosed with diabetes more recently. Most were diagnosed when they sought medical care for an acute event that brought them into the hospital. Despite living with the diagnosis for fewer years, lower-income individuals reported more depressive symptoms and diabetes complications, suggesting that they may have had the condition for much longer. Putting off seeking care for unfamiliar symptoms may be a result of mistrust of medical care in the first place, but in many cases women described prioritizing other family members' needs over their own. It may also be assumed that families residing in the lower-income neighborhood had less exposure to diabetes knowledge via public health messaging or simply by having community members with the condition. Lower recognition of the condition at the community level may have had an impact on self-care for diabetes by and in the family.

Yet, some women, such as Sarita, communicated fatalism toward their diabetes. Sarita was a middle-income woman with diabetes who described family conflicts as causing tension throughout her life, including with her husband and mother-in-law. Whenever she was blue, she read religious scriptures or slept; she didn't have many friends apart from her family. Even though her mother was diagnosed with diabetes at a young age, she knew little of diabetes at the time. She began to understand the condition only when she, her husband, and in-laws were diagnosed with it. Yet, Sarita described some apathy about her own diabetes—explaining that she rarely cared for her condition and ate whatever was put in front of her. This was somewhat surprising, given that Sarita had taken on the responsibility of caring for the diabetes management of many people in her family for many years. After those family members passed away, she took little interest in her own condition. These life stressors may have fueled her mild depressive symptoms. They might also have fueled her apathy toward her diabetes. However, she was concerned because both of her sons had been diagnosed with diabetes.

Why Gender and Family Matter

The narratives in this chapter show how different financial worries became manifest and imbued in syndemic suffering. The different ways in which social stresses materialized between men and women, wealthy and poor—from joint family stress to caregiving and personal health—underscores how gender and subjugation shift priorities and underlying causes of worry. These worries, which are inherently linked to gender and financial insecurity, influence how people experience the world and may be the cause of the elevated anxiety and depression found among people with diabetes in Delhi.[15]

In Delhi, the poverty-diabetes syndemic produces not only gendered subjectivities that impede women's physical health but also trans-familial suffering that poses challenges for mental health and caring for chronic illness. Thinking about diabetes across the social gradient within the context of globalization provides critical insight into how people may experience cultural change differently and how this may become reflected in the distress linked to diabetes. In this way, structural factors that affect the poor may not only be associated with financial insecurities related to food or housing but may also be mired in cultural expectations of dowries and marriage-linked social mobility. Moreover, trans-familial suffering within the diabetes experience may place an extraordinary burden on the women who care for those with diabetes and reinforce the subjugation of women who live with chronic illness. In this way, social interactions are coproduced within the family-disease nexus. Therefore, individual factors are somewhat sidelined within people's stories (and even more so among lower-income interlocutors), suggesting that social and psychological suffering may be more closely related to relationships within the family than to individual trauma.[16] Thus, my study in Delhi reinforces how fundamental an understanding of the family is for interpreting how individuals experience and perceive diabetes, distress, poverty, and social trauma.

4

SOWETO

Sibongile

A small woman with a round belly, wearing a turquoise blouse and tan pants, Sibongile appeared nervous and distracted when she arrived two hours late for our interview. We met at a research center, where for two decades she had participated in a cohort study located on the campus of the Chris Hani Baragwanath Hospital, or "Bara," Africa's largest public hospital. Bara was situated in Soweto, one of Johannesburg's largest and best-known townships. Sibongile was comfortable in the center, as she came by every year or so. Once we had a cup of tea and settled down in comfortable chairs, Sibongile relaxed and spoke for more than three hours, beginning with her childhood. Sibongile's story is a complicated one that brings to light some of the more visceral aspects of living life on the margins in a South African township.

Sibongile was born in a rural part of KwaZulu-Natal, a province hugging the coast of the Indian Ocean. Her father left when she was a young

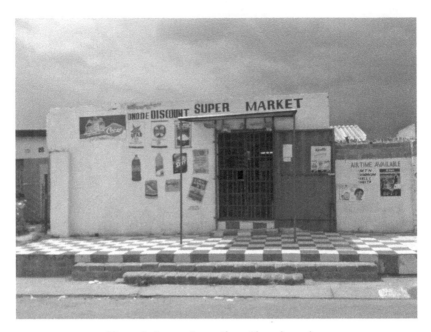

Figure 6. Soweto Spaza Shop. Photo by author.

girl, and she grew up with her mother and stepfather (although they never legally married). Her mother worked as a housekeeper for a wealthy white family and resided on the premises. Sibongile resided alone with her stepfather, who sexually abused her frequently between the ages of ten and sixteen; when she complained to her mother, Sibongile painfully recalled, "My mother would get upset and punish me and I would stop. I told my mother that I wanted to move out the house and go back to the homeland where I was born." For many years, however, Sibongile could not leave.

When she was seventeen, Sibongile met her first husband while visiting an aunt in Johannesburg. She never returned to her stepfather's home. She became pregnant with her first child soon after and married in haste. Yet Sibongile faced many unforeseen troubles with her marriage. She was dedicated to her husband but conflicted, stating, "My marriage was not easy for me." She explained, "I found out soon after I got married that my husband had epilepsy and it was a huge shock to me. Nobody had ever told me about that and it has caused me a lot of uneasiness. Each time that I'm away, I worry about him."

Sibongile served as mother and primary breadwinner for many decades. She worked in a factory to financially support her husband, two daughters, and her eighteen-month-old granddaughter who resided in her home. She also served as caregiver to her husband and children. She described her life as "a constant battle" and said that she worked so hard simply "because I'm forced to work to feed the family." With the help of her husband's small pension, she usually could pay for her family's immediate needs. Nonetheless, she complained of an outstanding debt that she must repay from a period when she was out of work. This compounded the fact that she felt stressed by living in an informal settlement within Soweto in which she described feeling "insecure." She explained that she applied for a low-cost home or "RDP house" associated with the government's Reconstruction and Development Program but had not yet been selected. This program "was aimed at eradicating shacks in Soweto but that hasn't been successful yet." The insecurity of her housing situation affected her everyday life, as she stated: "The place is not safe really. One has to always make sure that the doors are locked."

Later on, I asked Sibongile if she had ever faced burglaries in her home, as she had described feeling unsettled walking alone at night in her neighborhood. Sibongile's response surprised me, because none of the other participants who had described feeling unsafe in their homes or neighborhoods had reported anything so extreme. I sat quietly as Sibongile replayed this traumatic time in her life, providing much more detail than I expected:

> I had to install burglar guards [in my home] to prevent *tsotsis* [gangsters] from coming inside my house. There had been many robberies in the past. The first time they took my television set, the second time they raped my children. My children were raped before they had their own kids. While I was away they took some food, clothes and shoes, they took my eldest daughter's leather jacket as well. My daughter had just come back from a wedding and had valuables on her and they took everything off of her.

She paused before adding, "As my children grew up, it was not easy to find social workers. And reporting the matter at a police station could turn one into a laughing stock." After another brief pause, she continued with a softer, glummer tone: "I can't be happy like everybody else, when I go back home all the stress comes back. I get stiff shoulders and neck from the tension and sometimes I can hardly walk or move my arms." By pointing to the areas that got tense in her body, she physically located where she held stress and what somatic pain emerged. She went on:

> I do get support from doctors at times and they tell me not to worry about the problems I have. The last time he asked me what it is that was stressing me over the last couple of days and I told about this and that and that my husband was sick. He insisted that those were not new problems and I had to try and let go of them, not worry myself to death. Yet I find it hard not to think about them. I asked him, how is it possible that I stop thinking about my problems? These are within my system.

Sibongile and others used a common cultural idiom of distress, "thinking too much,"[1] to describe how she ruminated on her problems and held them close, including powerful emotions such as anger. In this way, her emotions were embedded in one another, with an increasing severity. She explained, "I'm not sure how to separate depression and stress." She connected stress with experiencing death in the family or something else that makes you feel down or rattles your core through the pain of losing someone. Stress, however, was related not only to emotional experiences but also to persistent financial problems. She said, "As a woman, I feel that stress is caused by the living conditions in my house."

Sibongile's stress also incorporated gendered notions of domestic housework and caregiving. When she began thinking too much, Sibongile often diverted her attention to "focus on other things" and "keep busy with house chores." She explained that she would often "talk to other people to try and let go of my troubles." She took a moment of silence and deep breath before she continued, "but it's hard." Like many women in Soweto, Sibongile relied extensively on her religious practice and religious community for strength during difficult times. When she felt stress, she explained, "I pray and put all my troubles to God because He knows all." Despite her impenetrable faith, Sibongile's thoughts continued to contribute to her thinking too much, causing ruminations and anxiety. She explained, "I sleep, but hardly fall asleep because my mind is always preoccupied." She went on—as many people did—to spin it positively. Sibongile smiled slightly and described an inner strength that was so common among my interlocutors: "I am grateful that I still wake up every morning and I still get that little sleep to stay sane."

Stress also manifested somatically. Sibongile described ulcers that she deemed "were caused by the fact that I had to look after my husband when I was still only a kid myself and I cried a lot." She made similar links to her diabetes: "My husband's health and situation could have been the causes of my diabetes." Sibongile also feared the consequences of these compounded health conditions. She stated, "I know there is a sickness in me and it can kill me anytime." However, she did not let these problems demoralize her; instead, she used illness strategically for self-care. She stated, "I can still do anything." Sibongile put her struggles in a positive light: "Diabetes changed my life because when I'm at work I feel tired and I need to rest. If I was home then I would use that time to properly sit down and rest. I constantly check the time to know when it is tea break or lunch time so that I can go to the toilet."

Sibongile's job at the factory afforded her consistent medical insurance, and so I asked her if she spoke with her physician about her stress. She said she had done so, but "I don't think he took it seriously." She felt that her physician was somewhat patronizing, telling her that she should stay busy and "avoid thinking too much." The physician explained that "keeping busy would get me very tired and sleep would come easier." She was confused by the notion that she should keep busy: "I always have things to do, preparing for work, cooking, and many other things."

Sibongile's determination likely played an important role in controlling her diabetes. She said that she received from the newspaper most of her information about what foods to avoid and how to prepare healthy meals for people with diabetes. She continued to "use a little fat when cooking" but stopped "frying food like meat, cabbage, [and] potatoes," preferring the grill. She noted that sometimes it was difficult to pay for some of the foods the physician recommended, but she strived to do so.

Near the end of our discussion, I pivoted to inquire how Sibongile perceived HIV/AIDS to have influenced her personal and medical experiences. Sibongile communicated one of the most nuanced understandings of what it was like to experience diabetes in the time of AIDS in Soweto. Sibongile, like most, had lost someone close to her to AIDS, including an uncle, a cousin, and other extended family. She explained that some "family members [are] suffering from HIV and some have passed on. My cousin, whose mom raised me, died of AIDS and I saw her during her suffering." When I asked her if there were any similarities between HIV and diabetes, she located HIV in her social world, stating, "I think so. Someone said something about diabetes being a chronic disease like AIDS." What Sibongile said next, which resonated with the thoughts of many other women I interviewed, was the most surprising and perhaps concerning take on the social connection of diabetes and HIV. She explained:

> I overheard people saying that some people are afraid to say that they had HIV so they say they have diabetes as a means of hiding the stigma that comes with being HIV positive. According to them there is no difference between HIV and diabetes as they all get a person bedridden and using diapers. People collapse and die on a daily basis and I think that is a good way to go. I don't wish to be bedridden and to wear diapers and I am not even sure that there would be anyone to help me. I don't know when and how I will die. People die on a daily basis and they continue to contract HIV, diabetes, and hypertension at alarming rates.

Sibongile sat with her hands folded in her lap and a serene expression on her face. After three hours together, I turned the audio recorder off and moved to inquire about her psychological symptoms. Sibongile reported moderate depression. Thereafter, Sibongile sat quietly for a brief moment. As she rose from the table, she said she felt a weight had been lifted after sharing her story, as many other women did. I escorted her out of the research center and we walked together until we reached the main road; she waved to me as she hurried off to catch the bus.

Methods and Context

Sibongile and others' narratives were collected in Soweto, a prominent township, or neighborhood, on the southwest side of Johannesburg. The expansive land-locked city of Johannesburg is the largest city in South Africa, being home to the nearly eight million people residing in the greater region. Nested in the Witwatersrand, a nutrient-rich range of hills, Johannesburg was founded in 1886 to exploit its minerals, especially gold. In the early 1900s, an explosion of industrial opportunities, in the mining industry in particular, attracted many rural Black workers and increased urban Black populations by nearly 94 percent, drawing people from agricultural, rural landscapes into industrial, urban ones. Many of those who worked in the gold mines resided in Johannesburg proper, although most were evicted by the British in the early 1900s and relocated to segregated townships. A growing tension between Afrikaners (Dutch migrants who had moved there more than two centuries before) and rural Black residents festered in rural areas across the country, often over the property rights to arable land. Although the complexities of colonialism and ethnicity are beyond the scope of this project, the historical legacies of injustice that shaped culture, consciousness, and the movement to urban centers cannot be overlooked in this context.[2]

In the nineteenth century, many people left the rural areas to seek work in the mines around Johannesburg, and from 1886 to 1917 there was a swift forced relocation to the area now known as Soweto (although the area was not formally recognized by the municipality). After the flu epidemic of 1918, there was an arousal of civic consciousness about the plight of residents in the six townships that now make up Soweto due to the shocking number of people who died from the epidemic; the state's response was to initiate the first housing scheme, with 227 houses built within a three-year period.[3] Over the next several decades there was uneven development of housing, water access, electricity, education, and other core state amenities. The greatest growth occurred during World War II, bringing an influx of workers, families, and citizens that exceeded the number of accommodations in the city. Today, like in the past, the majority of the city's nearly 1.2 million residents are "Bantu" or Black, claiming a variety of linguistic and ethnic heritages. The political category of "Black"—although very common today—was a sociopolitical construct that incorporated multiple African ethnicities into one category for the purposes of subjugation during apartheid.[4]

With fear and racism deeply embedded in the halls of political power, apartheid formed in 1948 as a state policy meant to consolidate political exclusion, economic marginalization, social separation, and racial injustice in urban South African spaces.[5] In opposition to this, a collection of the *Southwestern Townships* known as "Soweto" formed in 1963 when numerous neighborhoods combined into one collective name. One of Soweto's most prominent moments was the Soweto Uprising in 1976. As a center of Black political power, Soweto served as a stronghold of political resistance to the apartheid regime. In 1976, riots erupted in response to the government's ruling to teach in Afrikaans (the language of many

apartheid leaders) in schools, as opposed to the students' native and preferred languages. These riots are known to have prompted the regime
to bring more electricity and amenities to Soweto and to have eventually contributed to the downfall of apartheid in the early 1990s. Today,
Soweto incorporates people representing multiple ethnicities, languages,
and histories, including IsiZulu, IsiXhosa, Setswana, Sesoto, and Xit-
songa. With its relative wealth, Soweto continues to be a major political
and organizing center with a well-established middle-class, large shopping mall, historical museums, and prominent residents, including the
late Nelson Mandela, who lived here for many years. This makes Soweto
different from many other townships where the residents are more commonly lower income and transient.

My research study was nested within a research station at Bara hospital in Soweto. The Imperial Military Hospital Baragwanath was built
in 1941 during World War II to serve as a British Military Hospital. The
world's third largest hospital, and Africa's largest, Bara sprawls across a
large campus and is publicly financed. It is a teaching hospital for the University of the Witwatersrand Medical School and others. One building on
Bara's vast campus is the headquarters of the Developmental Pathway for
Health Research Unit (DPHRU) at the University of the Witwatersrand's
Faculty of Health Sciences, which is where I was a post-doctoral fellow.
Although I often walked with women across the research campus and
through the hospital after our interviews, most of my time was spent lis-
tening to women's life stories at DPHRU. Most women sought care at
Bara or outlying community clinics, and only some supplemented this care
with visits to private clinics. All of them had received care from the public
system most of their lives.

The research from my post-doctoral fellowship was intended to unpack
the complexities of women's experiences living with diabetes in Soweto.
The women I interviewed had been enrolled as caregivers for more than
two decades in what is known as the Birth to Twenty Plus cohort study.
Birth to Twenty Plus is a longitudinal cohort study originally called "Mandela's Children" because the children who have been followed since 1990
were recruited soon after Nelson Mandela was released from prison.[6]
Birth to Twenty Plus is one of a number of longitudinal cohort studies
dedicated to investigating the Developmental Origins of Health and Disease (DOHaD), which supposes that gestational and early life nutritional

stress may be more powerful in predicting health and disease than genetics. Birth to Twenty Plus has followed the social and biological lives of not only children but also their caregivers, all of whom were Black South African. It is among this group of caregivers that I identified and recruited eligible women to participate in a smaller study of diabetes and social experiences.[7]

My interlocutors from Soweto represent the broader cultural and linguistic diversity of the ninety-four-square-mile area; they are unified by their resettlement in Soweto, long-term residence, and enrolment in Birth to Twenty. Among the more than 1,000 caregivers, only 73 women had been previously diagnosed with diabetes. My research assistant, Hunadi Shawa (who prefers to be called "Mama Hunadi") called every eligible woman, and twenty-seven agreed to meet with me. Most who did not participate were unavailable or deceased.

I met with my interlocutors in a small private room in the research station at Bara. I conducted most of the interviews myself and relied on Mama Hunadi, a multilingual research assistant who had worked for several years at DPHRU, to recruit eligible women and conduct six interviews in Sesotho or Zulu. Meikie Hlalele—a research assistant who had worked at DPHRU for many years—stepped in to help with the translation of two interviews when Mama Hunadi was unavailable. I observed every non-English interview, discussed each of these interviews in depth, and co-constructed the field notes with Mama Hunadi and/or Meikie after they completed the interviews in Sulu or Sesotho. After the interviewees provided informed consent, we spoke on average for two to three hours, including primarily a life history narrative interview[8] followed by the administration of the Center for Epidemiological Studies Depression Scale (or CES-D),[9] specific questions about sociodemographic data, and a self-report survey of previously diagnosed medical conditions.[10]

Sibongile and others were a small reflection of the larger Birth to Twenty cohort. All the women were more than forty years of age, and two were more than seventy. Most had less than twelve years of schooling, and many relied on monthly government pensions or less to meet their basic needs. Few had health insurance, and most sought care from public primary care clinics in their neighborhoods as well as Bara. Many women had had diabetes for more than ten years, and most had at least one co-occurring physical condition like hypertension, arthritis, and psychiatric distress. Although

HIV and tuberculosis are highly prevalent in Soweto,[11] none of my interlocutors described having the conditions. Yet, all women described being affected by HIV and losing one or more family or friends to the disease.

Most women described around five stressful experiences that were overlapping and interactive throughout their lives (figure 7). Some described how childhood poverty prevented them from completing their schooling, how child abuse or spousal abuse continued to persist in their memories,

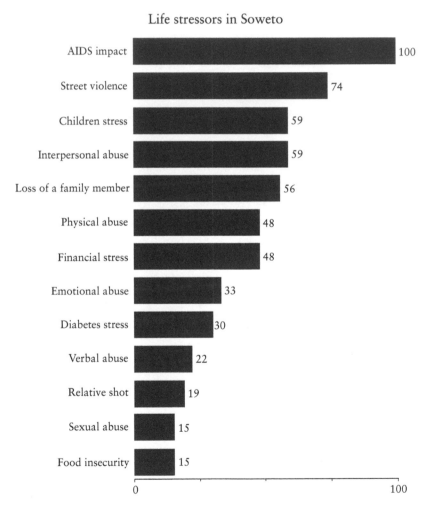

Figure 7. Life stressors in Soweto

and how financial insecurities continued to affect them throughout adulthood. Financial insecurity afflicted nearly everyone, interfering not only with their chronic illness but also, as elsewhere, with their family's needs and especially the need to meet social expectations or allow their children to complete school. Caring for their children, and in many cases their children's children, was a major worry for many women. These worries consumed not only women's time but also the finances that they might have used for themselves. Many women, like Sibongile, also described feeling uncertain or unsafe in their neighborhoods; they not only told their own stories but also spoke of the threat of what might happen or did happen (such as a relative being shot down the street many years before). The legacy of AIDS also emerged as a fundamental form of stress, associated not only with the loss of loved ones but also with the social and financial demands of caring for those they left behind.

Syndemic Suffering in Soweto

Syndemic suffering in Soweto mirrored syndemic suffering in Chicago in meaningful ways. Like in Delhi, many features of VIDDA emerged in Soweto, such as chronic poverty from childhood to adulthood, interpersonal violence and other social traumas, gendered expectations within the family, and overburdening expectations of caregiving. These individual-level factors can be situated within broader macro-social forces—much like VIDDA—that not only structured opportunities for men and women but also subjugated Black South Africans through colonialism and apartheid, physically segregating and systemically marginalizing them. In many ways, these forms of structural violence are embodied in diabetes; however, important cultural and social forces have emerged apart (though not dissociated) from such violence. These unique features differentiate Soweto from Delhi and Chicago in meaningful ways and exemplify how syndemics involve not only biological interactions between diseases but also social ones. Specifically, the stigma attached to AIDS and the fact that AIDS defined what it meant to live with a chronic illness shaped how people perceived diabetes, diabetes care-seeking, and diabetes stigma. Imbuing diabetes with AIDS had a major impact on how people reconstituted their identity post-diagnosis, which is inherently contextually mediated.

For Sibongile, being the sole financial provider and caregiver created extraordinary stress in her life. Living in an insecure structure also cultivated feelings of personal insecurity and hypervigilance that dated back (and perhaps beyond) an incident whereby her poor housing condition allowed perpetrators to break through and not only rob her but also harm her children. Having endured sexual violence during her own childhood, this incident with her children may have been particularly damaging (and remains seared in her memory). Sibongile could not disentangle the chronicities of structural and social problems from her persistent psychological and somatic symptoms, which would ebb and flow. Despite such challenges, Sibongile demonstrated personal strength by striving to eat well and manage her diabetes symptoms. This may be a reflection of her success at caring for her family for so many years: She always met the demands in front of her. Sibongile's commentary about how people perceived diabetes as a chronic disease like HIV points not only to the challenges of caring for diabetes but also to the social experiences of people facing a new type of "catch-all" chronic disease that conflated diabetes with HIV and its associated stigma.

The following analysis of syndemic suffering portrays how structural violence and HIV play complex roles in the way people come to embody and experience diabetes. First, the poverty and structural violence held over from colonial oppression and the apartheid era that marginalized people in Soweto and other urban townships were at the origins of the unequal distribution of infections and noncommunicable diseases like diabetes. Revealing how conditions like HIV and diabetes have become syndemic unveils how fundamental such oppression is in the affliction of disease. Second, the plague of financial insecurity contributed to women's "thinking too much," which manifested in worries from keeping a roof above one's family's head to purchasing fresh vegetables and fruits to adhere to the doctor's orders. Third, personal insecurities were integral to women's stories, from interpersonal violence experienced during childhood and early adulthood to feeling unsafe walking alone in their neighborhoods. Finally, AIDS-related social stigma around care-seeking for chronic illness fundamentally shaped how people experienced diabetes. This final point diverged from VIDDA, as did the fact that in many cases the types and clustering of social stressors women faced were somewhat more extreme. The rest of this chapter draws from interlocutors' narratives to consider how syndemic suffering in Soweto reveals both geographic vulnerabilities and a distinct local experience of stigma-by-association that fundamentally shape the social life of diabetes.

Geographic Vulnerability

Didier Fassin (2002, 2007, 2009) has argued that the structural violence instituted by colonialism and apartheid produced the profoundly negative impact of HIV and AIDS on Black South Africans, exemplifying the notion of geographic vulnerability. In *When Bodies Remember*, Fassin (2007, 24) describes one woman's protest of such inequality embodied in her life story, calling her story of AIDS not only a "biological state" but a "political fact." What Fassin (2009, 24) describes as an "ordinary existence" during a state of emergency in the township includes many of the experiences shared by my interlocutors, such as extreme poverty, physical insecurity (in the home and the street), absent and/or alcoholic parents, siblings killed by police, social marginality, lack of reward for school success (or no opportunity to finish school in the first place), and hopes for social mobility or emotional calm repeatedly destroyed. In many ways, HIV in the new democracy cultivated "new forms of violence" such as the shunning of neighbors, a government-imposed unavailability of therapeutic drugs, destitution due to reliance on state grants that are never provided, and medical care that is never realized.[12] Two decades later, the political realities of subjugation and marginalization of many of my interlocutors mirror the social and economic realities described by Fassin, while introducing new complexities like diabetes.

Nomfuneko exemplifies such complexities today. Nomfuneko spent her early years with both parents, but remembers constant discord; an early memory was being burned at the age of two because, as she recounts, she got stuck in the middle of her parents' fight. After her father died, when she was eight, her mother remarried, and her new father did not like Nomfuneko or her two siblings. Nomfuneko and her two siblings eventually left to live with her grandparents; she had minimal contact with her mother until she was an adult. Residing in a rural area under apartheid posed extraordinary stress: She had no money and only one dress that she had to wash herself. She persevered and eventually finished high school. In addition to experiencing childhood poverty, physical abuse, and emotional detachment from both parents, Nomfuneko was raped when she was seventeen. She explained that she didn't tell anyone because she thought nobody would care. After high school, Nomfuneko got a job and technical skills that commenced her independence. She soon married and had two daughters, although she separated from her husband after eleven years of marriage. Nomfuneko swept over that period of her life, dismissing it as "problems." She and her ex-husband still spoke about their children, and he had always provided financial support. When we spoke, Nomfuneko lived with both daughters in Soweto and spent her days caring for her eldest daughter's baby, who was six months old. However, she stated that she continued "thinking too much," mostly about the loss of her siblings: One was shot and the other died from "smoking" (i.e., cancer). She had not worked since her company went under in 1996, which caused persistent stress and financial insecurity. Soon after she lost her job, she was diagnosed with diabetes. Nomfuneko identified poverty and childhood trauma as the causes.

In many ways, AIDS represents the social and political inequalities of the apartheid era as much as diabetes reflects the stunted progress that followed it. In regard to AIDS, Fassin (2002, 64) contends: "If the epidemiological crisis in South Africa has no precedent, one should realise that, rather than being an exception, it is the most extreme illustration of the tragic link observed all over the world between the structures of societies and dynamic of disease." The emergence of diabetes amid inequality and structural violence reveals a contemporary story of suffering and social change. In some ways, diabetes among low-income Black South Africans marks the rapid social and economic changes that have accompanied the end of apartheid. This rapid change is visible in the building of modest new homes in Soweto as well as new shops and a modern mall, while many people remained employed but stuck in shacks like Sibongile's family, facing repeated barriers to social mobility (such as paying school fees). In part, the success of ART for AIDS in increasing life expectancy for more than a decade has played a role in elevating the number of people living with diabetes. There is also an important economic argument undergirding this problem, however, as economic development after apartheid has, despite overall growth, pushed the poorest households further into poverty.[13] For instance, within five years from the end of apartheid the poorest households' incomes went down.[14] With diabetes creeping into townships where the pocketbooks are not getting thicker, and in some cases are getting thinner, there must be a more complex interpretation for the rising cost of diabetes that moves beyond economic and social "progress."

Violence Embodied

Violence played both a visible and an invisible role in women's stories, and it manifested in syndemic suffering in three fundamental ways. First, structural violence contributed to hidden hungers that manifested in uniquely local forms of food insecurity. Hidden hungers reflect full bellies without substantial micronutrient diets, such as eating the traditional starchy staple pap (a thick porridge) until one is full, but abstaining from meat or vegetables due to the cost. This food insecurity mirrored what is often called a food desert in the United States, because the problem was not that people felt hungry (their bellies were full); rather, it was that they consumed empty calories like pap, or oily, salty, or sweet foods that were readily available and relatively cheap but not nourishing. Yet the idea of a food desert, initially proposed in the United States, as places in which fresh fruits and vegetables are hard to come by was not relevant in Soweto. The streets of Soweto are lined with informal stands selling fresh fruits and vegetables, where anyone can stop and shop as they pass by. Rather than lamenting access problems, many people stated that it was difficult to find the time to prepare these foods when delicious, cheap, salty fats were available on the go. One woman said, "Junk food is a common treat in the Township . . . [and] the order of the day, mostly during lunchtime. I have had to forego all of those, including those little chip snacks sold in plastics by most vendors." Most women made it very clear that what they were expected to eat according to the clinic was not possible in their kitchen. In most cases, this was because of cost. Many women repeated, "I do not have the money to buy the necessary food," and "I am not troubled much by being diabetic, save for the fact that I do not have the money to buy the food I need to eat. The right food is very costly."

The food desert that has been a subject of research and policy in the United States[15] does not easily translate to the urban South African experience. This is largely because, as Jane Battersby (2011, 550) argues, people depend on a cash economy, so "when income generating potential declines or food prices increase they become prone to food insecurity."

She emphasizes that because low-income urban communities have no "alternative sources of food," they are more food insecure compared to rural areas or wealthier parts of town.[16] The concept of urban "foodways"[17] further exemplifies this experience, highlighting that people do not depend exclusively on markets to purchase foods because, in some instances, they rely on neighbors or other family members when cash is unavailable. Battersby's (2012, 146) concept of "geographies of food retail" emphasizes the structural barriers, such as location and types of markets available (including *spaza* shops, which resemble US corner stores), that prevent people from having a diverse diet with limited sugars. This results in consumption of fats, sugar or honey, and meats (which are not helpful for those with diabetes), leading to full bellies and hidden hunger.[18]

Second, structural and symbolic violence were a fundamental part of women's narratives, blending sexism, racism, and classism in ways that limited their life chances. Most women were poor, including the more than half of our sample who relied exclusively on pensions of R1200 (around $136) per month to get by in Johannesburg. In some cases, these women's pensions supported their families, and in others they were supplemental income. For instance, one woman in her early sixties said, "I only make a few cents from the beadwork and I supplement that with the social grant that I receive from the government." Further, the social and economic impact of apartheid lingered in women's lives by putting economic barriers to completing school and forcing them to work at a young age, as exemplified in Nomfuneko's story. These systemic inequalities persisted long after apartheid, as demographic evidence suggests that women, and especially women of African descent, experienced more economic deprivation post-apartheid than men.[19]

Third, everyday violence was gendered and repeated throughout women's lives. Like my interlocutors in Chicago, three in five women in Soweto related some form of verbal, sexual, or physical abuse during their lifetime, and three in four reported some form of violence in the street (with one in five suffering from the loss of a relative to such violence). Sixty percent of women communicated some type of domestic violence, and for many this continued throughout their lives. The most severe prolonged violence was suffered by one woman who explained, "I have basically been abused throughout my life." These acts of aggression within the home that have become normalized and often hidden from view, such as child abuse in Sibongile's case or wife battering in many others, reflect broader social patterns of gender oppression linked to race and class. This trend reflects broader trends of female homicide, which afflicts mostly Black women: Violence by intimate partners in South Africa is six times the global average, and limited governmental resources are expended to mitigate this problem or support women and children who suffer from it.[20] Moreover, nearly half of deaths attributed to injury result from domestic violence—four and a half times the global measure.[21] The frequency and relative impact of intimate partner violence has been documented as well—often occurring not once, but repeatedly.[22] This form of constant, normalized stress in women's lives cannot be dissociated from women's psychological suffering, and it is reflected in the nearly half of women who reported depressive symptoms or the many women who described "thinking too much." Such memories of abuse were often the object of their ruminations.

Public acts such as street violence have also become normalized in Soweto. This was exemplified most powerfully in Sibongile's fear associated with past aggressions that were located in the street but transferred into her home. Three-quarters of the women interviewed reported violence in the public sphere—from burglary to losing a family member to gun violence—to be a central part of their lives. Almost every woman reported falling victim to violence associated with tsotsis, and many of these experiences were extreme. Pauline, for example, described the boys residing on her block: "I am scared of the young boys especially when they are under the influence of drugs. There is a new drug in town called Nyaupe, it is a combination of battery powder and crushed ARV tablets and they smoke them." She continued, "These children become so wild and out of control when under the influence of these drugs. Those are the kind of people who make me feel uncomfortable walking on the road and feel unsafe."[23] Male victims of homicide outnumber female victims 7:1, with men being the most common perpetrators and victims.[24] Thus, women not only feared what could happen or did happen to them but were also terrified of losing someone in their family, neighborhood, or church. Others lost their husbands to bullets during the apartheid struggle decades earlier.

As VIDDA illustrates, it is clear that such violence affects women's chronic psychological and physical suffering. Not unlike participants in

Chicago, most women in Soweto communicated how embodied violence was an underlying cause of somatic complaints, thinking too much, or diabetes. The social traumas at the center of women's narratives, by themselves or associated with other chronic and acute stresses, fueled the severe depression reported by nearly half of my interlocutors. Moreover, many women's distress was manifest in multiple morbidities—from diabetes to hypertension, cancer, stroke, and high cholesterol. With most women reporting at least one physical condition apart from diabetes, it is not surprising that they were so distressed. In a separate analysis of the whole cohort of caregivers from the Birth to Twenty Plus study, my colleagues and I found that psychological distress escalated dramatically when people had two, three, four, or more medical conditions.[25] This does not discount the impact of social trauma on psychological suffering; rather, it further demonstrates how intimately tied social stress can be to the mind and body.

Gender, Caregiving, and Diabetes

The social costs of losing loved ones and providing care in the midst of the AIDS epidemic were often hidden in plain sight. Losing someone they loved deeply caused extraordinary stress in many women's lives; the most common social cost, however, was caregiving for those left behind when their children died or left and their grandchildren became orphans. The situation is exemplified in the following exchange with Rachel:

> Rachel: The oldest grandchild is twenty-two years old, the second
>   born is twenty years, and the last one is ten years old.
> Emily: And where are their parents?
> Rachel: Their parents have passed away.
> Emily: How did they pass away?
> Rachel: They fell sick with AIDS.

Some women lost children and spouses to other causes, too, such as "heart trouble," "kidney problems," or "violence."

Moipone, for example, is the caregiver for three grandchildren whose parents died of AIDS in 2006. She was at first reluctant to speak about it. After her daughter died, Moipone was devastated and sought counseling for her grief. The demands of taking on the care of her three grandchildren, however, caused her to heal and find some balance in her life. After serving as their caregiver for six years, Moipone explained in the interview that the eldest—her twenty-two-year-old grandson—was the most stressful thing in her life. He went out at night, came home late, and spent time in the wrong crowd. Mostly she feared the night because, as with many women, she imagined that this was when most people would rape, kill, and shoot others. Moreover, her grandson often walked far from home to go dancing. This made her extremely anxious and caused her to lose sleep. She was grateful for her second grandson, who simply played basketball and swam with his friends. They were very close, and she felt calm about that.

Moipone was financially independent and demonstrated an extraordinary strength. She worked as a milk merchandiser at the Pick' n' Pay (a common supermarket chain) and had a large network of friends with whom she spoke often. She had never married and had always made her own way financially. In describing her independence, Moipone revealed that she derived a great deal of strength and self-worth from her work. However, it is also clear that she worked because she had to in order to support her grandsons. Losing her daughter to AIDS clearly had an impact on how she perceived the social world; this even came to bear on her conflation of HIV and diabetes. Her independence was also clear in how she frequented the public clinic in her neighborhood, as many of my interlocutors did, and would go once per month to have her blood pressure checked and her glucose measured. She always arrived at the clinic on time and had joined a group who met for social support to discuss their diabetes care, such as what foods to eat. Although few of her friends had diabetes and she was not sure why she developed the condition, Moipone was very much in charge of her diabetes and devoted to keeping her health.

Two in three women described how caring for children and grandchildren commonly caused stress in their lives. Most of these women, like Moipone, were primary caregivers to their grandchildren because their own children had died from AIDS, were in school, or were working full time. Some women lived with their children, like my interlocutors elsewhere, and therefore took care of their grandchildren during the day, like Nomfuneko. Others, like Moipone, worked to support their grandchildren in their children's absence.

Whereas Moipone demonstrated strength and independence in her diabetes care, many women grieved that their caregiving responsibilities impeded their diabetes care. One woman, whose daughter would abandon her children for long stretches of time, described feeling upset that her daughter would "just come and go as she pleased." This was in part because, as she stated, "I wasn't feeling too well myself as a diabetic. Sometimes I would have to be admitted in hospital and she would still be gone and the kids would be all alone forcing the older kids to forego school and look after the twins. I struggled to cope with the situation."

Better or Worse? Disentangling Diabetes from HIV

Due to the multiple forms of suffering in Soweto, where HIV and opportunistic infections like tuberculosis are common, it was difficult to ignore how other illnesses affected women's everyday lives. I explicitly inquired about perceived overlaps among diabetes, HIV, tuberculosis, and obesity, and I probed more after women described the complex social interactions between diabetes and HIV. Although most women identified a link between obesity and diabetes, or HIV and tuberculosis, the starkest results concerned the relationship of HIV and diabetes, as many women noted that "some people say that diabetes and HIV are just the same thing." Others stated that HIV and diabetes revealed similar identifying symptoms, such as Pauline: "Diabetes and HIV-positive people both get a runny tummy and loose stools and I get some kind of rash on my chest area whenever my sugar level is high, and HIV positive people have the rash on their chest." She went on to explain that this association was confirmed in her biomedical interactions: "I even asked a nurse who assured me that some symptoms are common in both ailments but I shouldn't worry myself much."

The longevity of the two conditions—which often last for life—was one of the most powerful connections that people made between diabetes and HIV. For instance, many described resemblances among the diseases because they both required treatment compliance for the rest of their lives. One woman stated: "I feel they are related, because with diabetes if you don't take medication you will die, and also with HIV if you don't take your medications you will die."

What was most surprising was that some women described HIV as being *better* than diabetes because of the better access to treatment. Flory, for example, stated, "I think that HIV is a better predicament compared to diabetes." She went on to explain that HIV is an easier condition to manage compared to diabetes: "Sugar diabetes requires more attention and there are certain foods that you have to forgo as a diabetic, unlike the HIV patients who just need to stick to their treatment and can still eat anything; better yet they can still recover and be like any other normal person." In this way, Flory made it clear that it was the change in food practices and the social dynamics of self-care that differentiated diabetes from HIV. She added, "Regardless of how faithful you are to treatment and diet as a diabetic, it still attacks you when you least expect it." This indicates that she perceived diabetes as something that was unknown and uncontrollable. Another woman suggested that diabetes was worse than HIV not because it was unknown, but because of the hard work required for self-care, stating, "Diabetes is worse than AIDS because it requires a lot of adjustment and management; you have to eat healthy and look after yourself and you have to exercise."

However, those who had close relationships with people with AIDS saw the two diseases as very much distinct. Maureen, for instance, explained: "People think that HIV is better than diabetes. I personally think that diabetes is better because one of my kids died of HIV and I saw her condition and it was really horrible how thin she was because of the disease. Most people I've seen who have the disease really get worse with it, and I don't think diabetes is worse than HIV." She went on to explain that she also knew people with diabetes: "My neighbor died of diabetes, but he looked very healthy and it was a Saturday and he had just come home from work. He went to the clinic and was referred to Bara after being diagnosed with diabetes, but he later died after a few hours. HIV really eats you up and by the time you pass on it would have been a long time coming."

Maureen's comments reveal what is at the heart of diabetes emergence in Soweto: the unknown. Despite the fact that Birth to Twenty Plus found that half of their cohort met the requisites for obesity and 14 percent were insulin resistant,[26] people remained less familiar with the condition. This is in part because people may not know they have diabetes, even if they are insulin resistant. In many cases, people receive a diagnosis only when they become sick and seek care. Thus, many of my interlocutors gathered information from personal experiences to interpret how diabetes might

affect them and their family members. This is also why the everyday inter-
ruption of diabetes self-care disrupts normal life, and therefore it explains
why diabetes is, in the eyes of some, worse than HIV.

Catch-All Stigma

The way people conflated HIV with other chronic diseases introduced a
surprising twist to their perceptions of and experiences living with diabetes. Anna explained, "A lot of people believe that HIV-positive people
prefer to say that they are only suffering from diabetes," noting that such
belief was culturally scripted and communicated in religious circles. Anna
regularly sought diabetes care and therefore received education about the
disease and how to care for it from the clinic at Bara. Anna was deeply religious, however, and put more trust in the information about health and
sickness she received from her pastor than in the instructions she received
from health care workers. She explained that the pastor argued that diabetes and AIDS were the same sickness, as demonstrated by our exchange:

> Anna: They say these sicknesses are the same. So they say we
>   shouldn't look at this any differently. According to them HIV
>   is no different from any other disease. Is there any truth to
>   that?
> Emily: Do they say that HIV is a sickness like diabetes?
> Anna: Yes, they do say that. They also say that it is also the same
>   as cancer. I think they are trying to discard discrimination
>   against these different diseases.

She alluded to the fact that her pastor meant to destigmatize HIV by
stating that all chronic illnesses were equal; therefore, Anna emphatically
repeated that she believed diabetes and HIV to be the same.

Others explained that people used other chronic illnesses, including
diabetes, to convey their need for regular medical treatment while al-
leviating HIV stigma. This social cost of self-care or medication seeking
was evident in women's narratives about routine medical care for diabetes. Some indicated that people associated routine medical care for diabetes with the routines of an HIV-positive patient, thereby inextricably
linking the diseases. In this sense, because of this association with HIV,

revealing one's need for daily medication and routine care produced unforeseen stigma not previously observed.

In some ways, this finding aligns with what was observed in the early days of ART. Early ethnographic accounts of the AIDS epidemic suggest that people abstained from speaking about HIV or any kind of terminal illness,[27] and that HIV treatment was often sought quietly, often relying on NGOs as well as the love, support, and generosity of family and friends.[28] Since those studies, ART has become widespread in biomedicine as well as in everyday speech. For example, a discourse analysis about how people spoke about HIV and AIDS suggested that people were attempting to normalize HIV and AIDS in everyday speech,[29] and that such normalization derived from the widespread use of ART in the most afflicted communities, like Soweto.[30] Anna's and others' narratives suggest that this work to normalize HIV may have had the unintended consequence of stigmatizing other conditions akin to HIV.

This produces what I call a "catch-all" chronic illness stigma that encompasses all chronic conditions requiring routine medical care. On the one hand, people with diabetes might be stigmatized because others assume they have HIV; on the other hand, people with HIV may use diabetes or other chronic diseases as a way to "pass" and avoid HIV stigma (for example, when someone says they "only have diabetes"). This conceptualization of a catch-all stigma category was perpetuated by social discourse, such as in the words of Anna's pastor.

In many ways, Erving Goffman's (1959) original conception of courtesy stigma is relevant to how women in Soweto conflated diabetes with HIV. Goffman's original explanation of courtesy stigma discussed how people became targets of stigma-by-association when their family or acquaintances were infected by a stigmatized disease. What my interlocutors in Soweto described, by contrast, is a different form of stigma-by-association, which is not between people but between diseases. Here, the courtesy stigma is the stigma attributed to regular care-seeking as a result of living with most chronic diseases. Catch-all stigma arises because the symptoms and care-seeking patterns for a chronic disease like diabetes closely resemble the symptoms and care-seeking patterns for HIV. This makes the stigma associated with diabetes almost undistinguishable from the stigma associated with HIV.[31]

Why Local Experience Matters

Rooted in a history of apartheid and AIDS, syndemic diabetes in South Africa portends a critical social and political-economic progress that has not been achieved. Women's stories reveal how the historical legacies of apartheid and AIDS continue to afflict their life chances as well as their everyday lives. Although women demonstrate at times extraordinary strength—in many cases serving as breadwinners and/or primary caretakers for multiple family members—the burden of those responsibilities becomes realized in their thinking too much, somatic pain, or diabetes. Many also described how letting go of their worries was the only way to stay healthy, while describing how deeply they felt the stress within their bodies. These common themes emerged across all narrative contexts—from Chicago to Soweto. What was most divergent and contextually rooted syndemic suffering in Soweto was a distinct cultural perception of diabetes. Conflating diabetes and HIV reveals how the social life of one disease can make an extraordinary impact on the social life of another. In some ways, the social life of AIDS has transformed the social life of diabetes, and it carries weight in what has become a double bind of chronic illness.

Thus, catch-all stigma played an important role in syndemic suffering in Soweto. Although many features of syndemic suffering may resemble VIDDA, imbuing diabetes with HIV stigma changed how people understood and experienced the condition. This was not different from the way diabetes was somewhat normalized in Delhi (albeit in an opposite direction). The attempt by the faith community to destigmatize HIV by linking it to other chronic conditions exemplifies what Arthur Kleinman (2010, 1518) has called an "unintended consequence of purposive (or social) action," as this framing passed the stigma from one chronic condition to the other. Initially hidden from view, these chronic conditions have now become epidemic and are in the process of reconfiguring not only new medical demands to care for an increasing number of people but also social demands. These social demands require careful education and policy interventions that recognize how people perceive diabetes and that do not further stigmatize them. Within a new social reality in which HIV and diabetes are intimately connected, syndemic suffering cannot be dissociated from the stigma of HIV or the historical legacy of apartheid, as those most afflicted face a confluence of old and new.

NAIROBI

Kandace

Kandace, a fifty-three-year-old woman of Nubian descent, was born and raised in the Kibera slum in Nairobi. Her parents farmed vegetables and potatoes on unoccupied lands to sell at the market, although they made very little money. Because she was their only child, however, her father wanted her to go to school and sent her to Nakuru, a medium-size city not far from Nairobi, to reside with her aunt and attend school. This was a very sensitive subject for Kandace, and she continued to look at her hands and speak softly as she shared this intimate story from her childhood. Kandace quietly recalled, "She did not take me to school. She just let me stay at home and work as a house help. She also maltreated me by beating me up whenever I asked her to take me to school." Kandace left this situation only when her father came to check on them when her aunt fell sick; she "started crying" as soon as she saw her father and told him that she "had never been taken to school" and asked him "never to leave me behind, and early the following

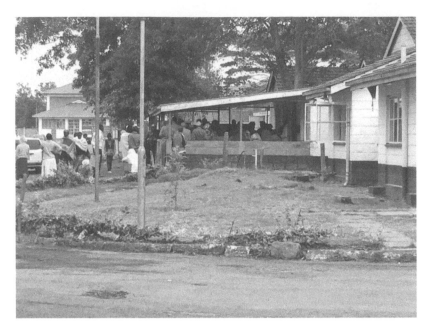

Figure 8. Waiting for the diabetes clinic at the Mbagathi District Hospital.
Photo by Author.

morning I left that house with [him]." She went home for a short time and eventually moved in with her grandmother, and she explained to Edna longingly how she "did not go to school" then, either.

Kandace said she settled in Kibera a "long time ago, when people were getting land for free." Her house and others were "all made up of mud," and she described many of her neighbors as "old people [who] depend on their children. Their children are the ones who work and therefore they spend time at home." Neither Kandace nor her husband worked in the formal sector, although her husband worked intermittently as a teacher. They had three grown children who resided in Kibera and were married, "apart from one who lives near me. I also live with my grandchildren and they [go to] school in Kibera. My children are still looking for jobs. One of my daughters trained in plaiting people's hair and she does business at the door stoop." However, the relationship with these children, as Kandace alluded throughout her story, was somewhat rocky.

There were also social and political tensions that bubbled beneath the surface of her environment and were central to her story. Kandace spoke of the land tensions that continued to persist in Kibera, often spurring ethnic conflict and at times violence, for example between Nubians and Kikuyus. Living in a mixed ethnic neighborhood, Kandace noted that there was ethnic tension that could at times be hidden. She explained, "Someone might say that they like you but maybe inside their hearts, they hate you. Even if you know that the neighbor is not a good person, there is nothing I can do about it." Kandace continued to describe Kibera as an insecure place, stating "there are theft cases everywhere in Kibera. . . . There are young boys who steal in Kibera. They also hijack vehicles and *matatus* [small buses] at night. These boys walk in groups and it is very difficult to know who is good and who is bad." She went on to say that she feared shootings and felt threatened in her neighborhood.

After describing some of these public experiences of fear, she circled back to her personal experiences. Although she had explained initially to Edna that she had a relatively civil relationship with her husband, Kandace dove into an intimate story that caused her extraordinary pain in her marriage, linking the onset of diabetes to her marital stress. She began, "You see, even my diabetes I think it came up due to stress." She described her husband's multiple "extra-marital affairs" with women in their neighborhood; in one case, "This was arranged by his relatives." She went on:

> But even before this happened, there was another woman in Kibera who came from Uganda . . . My husband started having an affair with this woman. He could leave as if going to the mosque and ended up sleeping in that woman's house. I never knew what was happening. After a short while, this woman was arrested over some issues and she was jailed. My husband and I started visiting this woman in Langata women's prison. I thought we were visiting a good neighbor, little did I knew that my husband was visiting his girlfriend. Sometimes I could even give my husband money to go and check on her.

Kandace went on to explain that her husband's relationship with this woman grew once she was released from jail, and eventually he moved in with her. She explained, "He reached a time that he was not hiding the act. He could go there in my presence. He moved there and started living with this woman. . . . When I confronted him and asked him, he mistreated me a lot. He went there and lived there. I think that is when my diabetes began due to stress. My husband was hostile to me, and he could not listen to me or even stay in my house." Eventually, however, "My husband came back to my house and apologized for what he did for me. . . . We now live together."

Kandace went on to describe stress as "thinking a lot, especially when I get angry." She said, "When my heart beats a lot, I also get tired and I have a headache. Generally, I usually feel my body aching. Even the story I have narrated to you, I became so thin that people started saying that I had AIDS. That was the thing that stressed me a lot. I sometimes felt like tearing a piece of cloth, I could just start crying a lot in a loud voice and so on."

Despite this, Kandace suggested that the only ongoing stress in her life was her diabetes. The stress was mostly associated with physical problems: "I have body aches and my eyes have a problem. My legs also sometimes become numb, especially when I stay without doing some walking as an exercise. I sometimes faint a lot." She also described, as many people did, how knowing someone with diabetes had an impact on her. She said, "Before I knew that I was diabetic, I had a neighbor of mine who is diabetic. She helped me a lot by referring me to a nearby clinic in Kibera where I went for diagnosis. When I went there, I was diagnosed with diabetes and my sugars were really high."

Kandace would often "cry and shout. I also pray a lot" to deal with stress. She described *huzuni*—a cultural idiom of distress roughly translated as grief—as a powerful feeling in her life.[1] She linked it specifically with the loss of a loved one, as many people do. However, Kandace also gave a broader meaning to it, which reveals how complex her emotions were around family and her health: "Huzuni is when you think a lot, especially due to death. Again, even when your own children desert you or hate you, you will feel huzuni. I have also told my husband never to shout at me due to my disease, because anything that causes me anger will make me have huzuni."

Like many, Kandace calls diabetes *kisukari*, or sugar. She was not sure how she developed diabetes but reported being diagnosed in 2008 at a clinic in Kibera. She said that she feels "nothing" when she thinks about diabetes. She went further: "Even right now, I will not feel anything even if you told me that I have AIDS, because once the disease has come into the body, there is nothing you can do." This fatalism accompanied her blank expression.

However, she described in depth how diabetes changed her life:

> If I don't walk I have problems with my legs. I can't work as much because I get tired easily. I also urinate frequently and if I delay going to the toilet, I usually have a problem. I can't even see well. . . . I feel so exhausted. When I asked the doctor about it, I was told that the insulin I use is affecting me because sometimes I inject myself without eating and that is how it affects me. I even can't travel because of how I feel like. I just want to sleep and stay in my house.

Kandace was adamant about the fact that she managed the disease herself. She did not feel alone, because many people in Kibera also had diabetes. Those people often went to the Wanga Clinic for care, but Kandace began going to Mbagathi for its specialty diabetes clinic, because the public clinics in Kibera "don't have insulin."

The cost of diabetes, however, created problems for Kandace and her family. She described how her vision was ailing her, but "sometimes I have no money. Again, I have been told to buy glasses for my eyes, but I have no money to buy the glasses." Financial insecurity was also linked to her skipping diabetes medications—in her case, insulin shots. She would often seek medical care at the larger hospital, which carried the medication she needed; if she could not make the payments, however, she would go to the local clinic "that gives medicines for free." She adhered to diabetes medications as closely as she could, but sometimes in the past she had skipped her medications to avoid their negative effects. She said, "Before, the insulin was affecting me and I used to skip injecting myself. But I have learnt that I must use it when I have already taken foods. Now, it is not affecting me as such."

Kandace was diagnosed with tuberculosis in the recent past: "There was a time I had diabetes and TB. But I knew why the TB came: I was building a house and the cement that was poured down affected me to get TB." She said she dealt with TB by taking her medicines: "I just took all the medicines as required and I got healed. What is important is to follow instructions when taking medicines."

She went on to explain that "all the other diseases can get into a diabetic person. Someone can also have asthma." Although she had many family members who were affected by HIV, which she described being like "the common cold," Kandace did not know anyone with HIV and diabetes. She explained, "HIV is a secret between the doctor and the patient. Many people nowadays hide their HIV and say it is diabetes."

At the end of the interview, Kandace was at ease and wanted to spend the rest of the afternoon sharing her life experiences. She chatted for a while longer before she headed back to the clinical room for her diabetes clinic. She slipped out the door after her clinical visit and nodded to Edna before she returned to her home in Kibera.

Methods and Context

Kandace's and others' narratives were collected in Nairobi, the capital city and the largest urban conglomerate of Kenya. Nairobi is situated right next to Nairobi National Park, a game reserve with a river running right through it. Nairobi is a green city, filled with public parks and forests and home to more than 6.5 million people from all reaches of East Africa—people from Western Kenya to the coast, as well as refugees and migrants from regional political hotspots such as South Sudan and Somalia. Founded in 1899, when the Uganda railway line was built for the British Empire, the city has a history of hyper-segregation, exemplified by the 1922 Vagrancy Act that segregated people by income, ethnicity, and economic identity. Known as "native reserves" in the colonial period, many slums today resemble those past efforts to enforce colonial segregation.[2] Kibera continued to expand as new residents arrived from rural areas and other neighboring countries; despite the critical housing situation, many of these residents had more pressing concerns than finding better housing, such as keeping their families afloat.[3] Today, Kibera epitomizes Nairobi's entrepreneurial spirit and aggressive politics as well as underlying ethnic tensions. These tensions surface at critical moments, such as during the presidential elections of 2008, but they often are hidden from view in the everyday life of urban and rural Kenya.[4] These tensions are not dissociated from the inequalities visible in Nairobi's segregated neighborhoods.

Kibera is Africa's largest slum and the most prominent in Nairobi. It was settled during the colonial era as an informal racially segregated settlement for returning Nubian soldiers, who were relegated to the periphery of the city after their service. These native reserves were physical spaces but did not permit land tenancy, something that has persisted for many families to the present day. Today Kibera remains an informal settlement owned by the government, formally acknowledged by it, and provided with political representation. Kibera has grown exponentially thanks to many African migrants who have moved to Nairobi to seek economic opportunities. Estimates of the population of Kibera differ—from 250,000 residents to more than one million—and the area shows huge ethnic diversity, including Luo, Luyia, Nubian, Kikuyu, Kamba, Kissii, and others.[5] The population of Kibera represents the socioeconomic diversity of Kenya, with middle-class families emerging among a majority of residents who survive extreme poverty, earning less than one dollar per day. This is physically evident in the houses that are packed together in Kibera, mostly small shacks made of wood with concrete floors that serve as home to around eight people. Most families are tenants with limited rights and difficult access to safe water, electricity, sanitation, jobs, health facilities, and secure homes.[6]

My research study was conducted at a public hospital clinic at Mbagathi Hospital, one of the largest feeder hospital clinics for the Kenyatta National Hospital. The Kenyatta National Hospital is the oldest hospital in Kenya, and it serves as a public, tertiary referral hospital for the Ministry of Health and a primary research and teaching hospital for the University of Nairobi. We consulted with their chemistry lab to analyze some biological data for the project. But Mbagathi Hospital is a much smaller facility and therefore serves fewer patients, most of whom reside near the clinic. Many people from Kibera seek medical care at Mbagathi simply because of its location and accessibility. Yet, the diabetes clinic is one of few such clinics across the city, so many of my interlocutors recruited at the clinic traveled there from low-income neighborhoods. Because of Kenya's two-tiered health system, with the public system serving as a safety net for more than half of the population, the Mbagathi Hospital sits only blocks away from a large private hospital.

The research I conducted in Nairobi was in collaboration with the Africa Mental Health Foundation (AMHF), a nonprofit research center dedicated to improving access to mental health care and knowledge about mental illness. Founded in 2004, AMHF involves multiple large projects that are focused on multidisciplinary perspectives on mental health, substance abuse, and neurological disorders, with a special dedication to piloting mental health intervention projects. My research was both nested within the broader mission of AMHF and set apart from it. My colleague Dr. Abednegu Musau worked closely with me on the project to establish a relationship with the administration at the Mbagathi Hospital so that we could invite people from the waiting rooms of primary care and specialty clinics to speak with us. I also hired three research assistants and spent two weeks training them on how to conduct ethnographic interviews that involved multiple steps and multiple hours. It would have been impossible to conduct these one hundred extensive interviews in three months without their hard work, dedication, and intellect.

Gitonga Isaiah, a trained nurse, served as the lead study manager, recruiting patients from the waiting rooms of the primary care clinic and diabetes specialty clinic; the two clinics were located in separate buildings, although some patients attended both. Gitonga spent a great deal of time explaining the study, administering informed consent forms, and scheduling a time for the interview (which was often on that day or the next). The final step involved drawing blood from our interlocutors and walking the blood samples over to the University of Nairobi's Chemistry Lab, situated next to Kenyatta National Hospital; once the results were available, Gitonga called each of our interlocutors to communicate them. Because of the cost of diabetes testing and medical care, receiving some health information free of cost was an enticement to participate in the study for some.

I also hired Edna Bosire, who completed a master's degree in anthropology, and Gregory Omondi, a nurse. They were attracted to the study because of the methodology—Edna because she wanted more training and experience in anthropological research, and Gregory because he was interested in a career in research. The team was incredibly engaged, and following Gitonga's work, Edna and Gregory would sit with our interlocutors for two to three hours; the interview included a few survey questions about the interviewees' places of residence, homes, and families, followed by a lengthy life history narrative interview that lasted around two hours, and sometimes longer. They also conducted depression and anxiety inventories and checklists of previously diagnosed health conditions and mental health care experiences at the end of each interview.[7]

We initially set out to investigate how men and women navigated chronic illness and how people with and without chronic illness perceived it. From the waiting rooms, we selected 50 men and 50 women; half were previously diagnosed with diabetes, and the other half turned out to be insulin resistant after we analyzed their hemoglobin A1c. In part, their interest in the study may have been because we were testing for diabetes— a medical test that many interlocutors could not afford and therefore put off. Most people had two or more health conditions in addition to diabetes, such as hypertension, depression, chronic pain, HIV, tuberculosis or other chest problems, and acute bouts of malaria and typhoid.[8]

Only two people approached by Gitonga declined to interview, saying they did not have enough time. Most were eager to participate, however, and the majority of the interviews occurred after people completed their health care visits. They spoke in a private meeting room in either clinic, or on busier days in a private tent situated near the periphery of the hospital's campus. The research team was on site every day for nearly three months. We included only adults who were over thirty, and some were in their late sixties. All interviews were conducted in Kiswahili and translated to English after Edna and Gregory transcribed them. These transcripts were analyzed alongside extensive field notes Edna and Gregory wrote about each interview, which I read as soon as they were available and discussed extensively with them. We had two-hour-long meetings every Friday afternoon to troubleshoot, discuss common themes, and have lunch together. I was on the hospital campus at the beginning and constantly in conversation with my research assistants via texts and phone calls, but once the study was underway I stopped by the hospital only once a week because my presence was more distracting to the patients and the medical staff than helpful to the research team.

Of the one hundred interlocutors involved in our study, two-thirds were fifty years old or younger and were born outside Nairobi. Half were Kikuyu, one-fifth were Kamba, one-tenth Luo, and the rest were Luhya, Embu, Kisii, Nubian, or others. Nearly all were ever married, three-quarters had more than two biological and/or adopted children, and many men had multiple wives. Around 65 percent of the women had completed primary school or less, compared to 40 percent of the men. Yet, more women (20 percent) had completed a technical or professional school compared to men (10 percent). Twice as many women as men reported casual or contract labor or being employed while receiving a pension. Most lived in a slum, but the sample showed a notable socioeconomic diversity: One-fourth reported having a private flush toilet in their home (signaling a higher-income status), and around half reported having a communal toilet (lower-income status).

Our interlocutors in Nairobi reported more social stressors than the participants in the previous studies in Chicago, Delhi, and Soweto; they reported on average seven social stressors, with women reporting up to twelve and men commonly reporting more than four stressors (see figure 9).

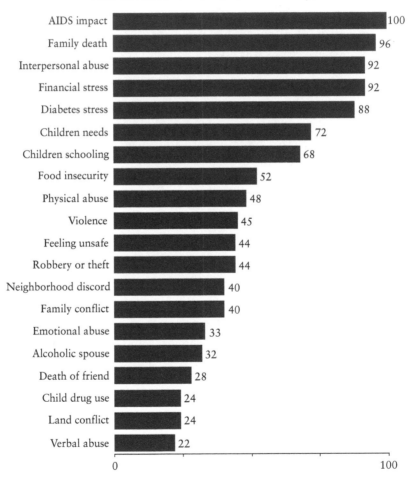

Figure 9. Life stressors in Nairobi (women only)

The worry about meeting financial needs was ubiquitous among both women (80 percent) and men (90 percent). In most cases, this included the burden of caring for children and paying for their schooling—or, as in Soweto, caring for those whose parents had died from AIDS or violence or had migrated for work. Interpersonal abuse was more common among women (84 percent) compared to men (40 percent), with most people citing verbal or emotional abuse and one in three citing physical abuse. Only four women mentioned sexual abuse. Family conflict was also extremely common, and in many cases it included land disputes related to inheritance. Finally, a feeling of insecurity was common, with many women having experienced some form of gang-related violence (either as a victim or an observer of gun violence, robbery, or other incidents). Figure 9 provides data about the association between stressors and diabetes for women in Nairobi, which can be easily compared with data in the previous chapters. Across the narratives from Nairobi, the ubiquity of HIV was similarly impactful on people's lives, but not necessarily in the same way it was in Soweto. The legacy of lives lost had a social and economic cost to those we interviewed; in many ways, people imbued perceptions of diabetes with long-held beliefs about HIV and AIDS. What emerged very starkly was a different economic impact of diabetes compared to HIV, which was intimately connected with health financing and international donor priorities.

Syndemic Suffering in Nairobi

Syndemic suffering in Nairobi mirrored syndemic suffering in Soweto in numerous ways, although there were significant financial and personal insecurities that created a more extreme experience among these interlocutors. Like elsewhere, histories of social and economic marginalization were pervasive in people's current realities in Nairobi. Like in Soweto, the social production of risk that emerged at the juncture of HIV and diabetes produced a unique landscape for identity work and social stigma around chronic illness. The most significant departure, however, was the more severe financial insecurity at home as well as within the clinic, which fundamentally shifted the experience and risk of diabetes in Nairobi. For example, the imposition of medical fees for diabetes care that did not exist for HIV care, a dynamic set by international donor priorities for infectious threats, had an unintended social impact on the way people prioritized diabetes in their own lives.

For Kandace, being ethnically Nubian and a practicing Muslim created a particular form of ethnic and religious marginalization. Despite the fact that Nubians are known as the original settlers within Kibera itself, they represent a much smaller portion of the population today (around 15 percent), with the majority of residents being Christian and belonging to various ethnicities, such as Kamba, Kikuyu, Luhya, or Luo.[9] Kandace's story reflects many of the major themes women in Nairobi communicated in their life history narratives: structural impediments such as limited schooling and financial insecurity, social struggles related to gender dynamics (in her case linked to marriage), and social exclusions. Kandace's childhood poverty introduced challenges that affected her throughout her life course, excluding her from a formal education and pushing her into an early marriage that led to an emotionally abusive life-long commitment. Significant undercurrents to her financial insecurity were the intergenerational obstacles to attain land tenure, ranging from her parents' farming on unoccupied lands to her claiming her current, long-settled home in Kibera as her own. These significant features cannot be dissociated from the way ethnicity is structured or from the complicated colonial and ethnic tensions that have perpetuated the marginalization of Nubians.[10] These feelings were further reinforced by her interactions with her neighbors. However, diabetes too played a fundamental role in causing her stress, and Kandace linked her chronic illness to her husband's infidelities. Yet, she did not deem diabetes to be a special condition—she noted that any chronic disease that makes one sick is somewhat irreversible, and she strongly believed that people must accept their fate. She ended on the note that diabetes itself is a complicated social experience because people often say they have diabetes to cover up HIV and stymie stigma. Comparing HIV to the common cold indicates how frequent such comparisons have become.

The following analysis of syndemic suffering shows how those diagnosed with diabetes in Nairobi negotiated financial insecurities inside and outside the clinic that shaped how they experienced, cared for, and perceived diabetes. First, structural violence became visible in the narratives of land grabs and displacement that were rooted in family conflicts and fostered deep-seated financial insecurities throughout the lives of many of our interlocutors. These insecurities manifested in stress associated with housing, children's expenses, and food—all factors that were intimately tied to living in low-income (and informal) settlements like Kibera. Second, personal insecurities played a role in Nairobi similar to other contexts, where sexual and physical violence were also common. In Nairobi it was surprising to find, however, that more people felt beaten down by verbal ragging compared to other contexts. Other forms of personal insecurities fostered people's hypervigilance in their neighborhoods, including the fear of gangs, gun violence, and robbery. Third, the compounded nature of these social stressors was unraveled in poor mental and physical health. The more social traumas people described, the more likely they were to report symptoms of depression, anxiety, and diabetes.[11] Finally, memories, experiences, and ongoing reminders of the HIV and AIDS epidemic persisted and defined how people perceived health or sickness and the everyday practice of seeking care. This was not different from what happened in Soweto, although the role of user fees in undermining how people thought about diabetes care was a defining feature of the narratives of Kandace, Ester, and others living with diabetes in Nairobi.

Violence, Land, and Insecurity

Regina's definition of mistreatment focused on a land dispute. When Edna asked her if she had ever been abused or mistreated, she angrily replied in the affirmative. She described a dispute with her "brothers and sister in Christ"—those who attended her church. She described how one brother in Christ lied to her and took a land title deed for his own gain. She had trusted this person to assist her with a serious problem (which was not discussed in detail), and he had asked her to give him the deed to serve as a guarantor for that problem. Regina immediately gave him the papers, and he eventually bribed an official and had the land title deed changed into his name. Regina later realized what happened and that she had lost her land worth 2.2 million Kenyan shillings (KES) (around $21,000). She was very upset; she explained that she had attempted to follow up on this grievance, but her old age would not allow her to move quickly. She went on to explain that these grievances were common for older women like her. For example, Regina reported the experience of a sister in Christ who had rushed to her house crying after having been thrown out for not paying rent. She pleaded with Regina to loan her 30,000 KES (less than $300) so she would not be thrown out of her home. She never repaid the loan. Regina said that she had forgiven her sister in Christ and did not expect to receive the money back; she explained that these things, however, had caused a great deal of emotional pain.

Feeling insecure in and about one's home was a powerful feeling across the four study sites, and it was most frequently repeated in Kenya. Whereas narratives that resemble Kandace's story illustrate how land tenancy may be rooted in colonial legacies and persistent inequalities, Regina's experiences reveal how squabbles over land can become a form of subjugation associated with gender or age. In Kibera, many people rent small shacks from others who do not necessarily have government rights to own the land.[12] The lack of the security and stability associated with home ownership is exacerbated by the abject conditions of these shacks along with the common reliance on communal pit latrines that, in many cases, are shared among numerous (one study noted as many as fifty) families.[13] One third of my interlocutors in Nairobi stated that they depended on these communal pit latrines.

Many also grieved the loss of rights to ancestral lands (often located in rural areas) due to myriad factors, including displacement, death of a husband, or the revoking of rights.[14] For instance, one woman said, "My brother in law abused me verbally after my husband's death. He wanted to grab land that was already given to me when my husband was still alive. . . . He took the piece of land that he wanted." Land grabs were not always gendered; as one man recalled, "They wanted to grab my piece of land. That's why I was even affected by diabetes. But finally I succeeded; they never grabbed it." For this interlocutor, the possibility of losing his home was felt so deeply within the body that he thought it had triggered his diabetes. These cases exemplify how tenuous living situations were for some interlocutors compared to those people who owned their homes and could enjoy a sense of security as well as several amenities.

Beyond this underlying financial uncertainty, personal insecurities in Nairobi mirrored those in Chicago, Delhi, and Soweto. It was somewhat surprising that sexual and physical abuse was found to be lower than in other studies in other contexts as well as other studies conducted among women in Kenya;[15] in some cases, what women reported in our small study was less than half of what was reported elsewhere.[16] When I discussed this with my colleagues at AMHF, they spoke to the fact that such violence had become so normalized that people might not report it as violence. For instance, my colleague said over coffee that child battering may be perceived to be discipline rather than abuse, and therefore it would not be reported as a mistreatment. This argument is unsubstantiated; however, it introduces the possibility that the way people perceive interpersonal abuse likely influences their reporting of it in a once-off interview, as well as their interpretation of the experience as destructive or normative. Conversely, the frequent reporting of emotional abuse or verbal ragging in this study indicates that interpersonal torment unnerved many people. In many cases, a family member (often a parent or spouse) or someone residing in close proximity to the victim perpetrated verbal ragging as well as other forms of abuse.

Feeling insecure within the public sphere was also as common in Nairobi as it was elsewhere. This was in part due to the pervasive threat associated with gang activity and lack of police representation and protection.[17] For instance, one man said, "There is no security; if you are late you will definitely be mugged"; another stated, "There are a lot of theft cases, gun shooting, and all these make us live in fear." One-quarter of our interlocutors reported feeling unsafe, for example by noting that "there is no security" and "sometimes you are robbed by force; they come to your house and demand things and it could be worse if you don't give them, so you are forced to comply." The salience of gangs in informal settlements like Kibera cannot be dissociated from the high unemployment and limited economic opportunities among young men in this context. With nearly half of the sample describing feeling unsafe due to gun violence, neighborhood discord, and robbery or theft, it was clear that hypervigilance was pervasive. This cannot be dissociated from mental health in the short or long term, and it may even play a role in metabolic disturbances like diabetes through a link to inflammation.[18]

Gender, Caregiving, and Diabetes

Financial concerns related to caring for children—such as keeping clothes on their backs, food in their bellies, and their school fees covered—were common threads opined by men and women alike. Caring for orphans of family members who had passed away due to AIDS was not uncommon in Nairobi, reflecting findings in Soweto. In both cases, the financial demands of caring for children were given priority over the health needs of our interlocutors, who were very dedicated to their families. In many cases, healthy foods that catered to the needs of people with diabetes were outside the purview of the family due to cost. Food insecurity reflected the challenges with food access in Soweto, but it was compromised further by the escalation of the costs for foods and fuel linked to rapid economic growth in Nairobi.[19]

These problems were exacerbated among those who navigated the poverty-diabetes nexus. Nearly half of the women and one-fifth of the men reported food insecurity. It was interesting to find, however, that men with diabetes were least likely to describe feelings of food insecurity, which may reveal a gendered injunction to prioritize care for the patriarch within the family (in this as in many other male-dominated societies). When asked whether diabetes had changed her life, one woman responded: "A lot, because I used to buy food that would take us the whole month. But with diabetes, it needs a special diet, something that has constrained my budget. It is hard for poor people like us." The problem, however, was not only food. Many with diabetes described the pressure to exercise regularly and meet the dietary expectations of clinicians to be stressful. David, a forty-year-old man with diabetes, described this problem very clearly: "It is not a diet that you can just pop into any hotel. It's not something that you can just order and just be brought on the table. So you have to organize yourself. You have to take a good meal. . . . The diet for diabetics is a bit expensive." This quote exemplifies how nutritional advice for someone with diabetes is not only out of the ordinary for someone living in Kibera but also out of reach.

These factors interwove in important ways. Grace, for example, was a sixty-four-year-old grandmother from central Kenya who supported fifteen grandchildren financially because their parents could not care for them. Some grandchildren came to stay with her after being displaced from Eldoret due to political violence. Grace explained that their parents found Nairobi to be a safer option for their children (although the parents remained in Eldoret). One of her sons, his wife, and their children resided with her because they were HIV positive and were taking ART;

she said that they were not able to care for themselves financially. Grace described having to work harder to earn more money to buy them food. Because she had so many mouths to feed, Grace could not afford school fees for all fifteen grandchildren, and many of them had to take extended breaks from school to save money. This was hard for her because it reminded her of her own childhood, when she could not attend school due to cost. Despite these stresses, Grace was dedicated to caring for her family and felt indebted to them because they had protected her from her brother-in-law who had tried to "grab" her land after her husband died from diabetes. It was after his death that Grace found out about her own diabetes, or kisukari (sugar). Purchasing the foods recommended by the clinic was almost impossible for Grace. Because the medication was too expensive, she often skipped it. She also frequently missed trips to the clinic at Mbagathi because bus fare was too costly. The stress of meeting these basic needs caused what she called a "pounding heart" and "constant headache."

It should not be surprising that the more social trauma and financial stress people described through their stories, the more likely they were to report somatic and psychological symptoms of depression and anxiety. In many ways, women's narratives demonstrated how their unequal social burden affected their social lives, economic decisions, psychological wellness, and somatic symptoms. Compared to men, women reported higher rates of anxiety, depression, financial insecurity, death in the family, abuse (in every subcategory), food insecurity, experience with robbery and theft, family conflict, unsafety, neighborhood discord, land conflict, pressure (meaning hypertension), alcoholic spouse, death of a friend, other violence, and children's drug use. This list accounts for sixteen of twenty (80 percent) stressors described by my interlocutors,[20] not including subcategories of abuse or diabetes-specific categories such as exercise and eating right. These gendered social inequalities shaped women's everyday lives and cannot be divorced from their psychological and physical suffering.[21]

Taking a close look at the differences between men's and women's health burdens also provides an important perspective on the gendered dimensions of their suffering. Compared to men, women reported more obesity, undiagnosed diabetes, uncontrolled diabetes, and comorbidities. Not only were most women overweight or obese, but many women (56 percent) without a previous diabetes diagnosis also were insulin resistant, and most with a diagnosis had poorly controlled diabetes. These data support other studies demonstrating that mental health is associated with obesity,[22] diabetes,[23] and multimorbidity[24] in women. This may be further compounded by the social roles that women perform within the family, often putting others' needs before their own, for example in the preparation of food. Such experience found in Nairobi closely mirrors what I found across study sites. Nevertheless, this does not detract from the unique social experiences of men and their suffering or tendency to stuff emotions through substance abuse, especially of alcohol and tobacco.[25]

Convergent Conditions

Hope described how complex someone's medical condition can be. "I have diabetes," she said; "I also have HIV. I have pressure. Of the three diseases, pressure is disturbing me. It has refused to go down." Hope and Esther (whose story opened the book) were the only two women with diabetes who also had HIV, although it was blood pressure that really bothered Hope. She went on to describe how being sick affected her social and financial life:

> I was admitted in the hospital for two weeks and I just asked the doctors to discharge me because I told them that many people depended on me. And by being in the hospital, I could not stop thinking on how my children were suffering. My pressure could not go down. My heart beats a lot even when I walk on a short distance. Even today when I came to the hospital my pressure was at 200 [mm Hg]. The doctor was shocked about that. This pressure is making me tired and fatigued. Sometimes I can't even hold a cup, it may fall down.

Many others connected diabetes and "pressure" in part because hypertension and diabetes are common companions. Many also linked these with other chronic conditions, for example by noting, "My body is not good, it aches a lot. This has affected my work. I have pains all over my body, especially my hands and legs." Many people also identified stomach ulcers and other somatic conditions. Unsurprisingly, this was commonly linked with social stress and psychological distress.

The connections with common infections such as tuberculosis and HIV reported by those with diabetes raised complex questions. Kandace described living with tuberculosis and diabetes for some time, although her tuberculosis was healed after she completed the treatment (which was provided free of charge and was prioritized by international donors). Another woman said she had a neighbor with tuberculosis and diabetes who successfully finished her tuberculosis treatment but never took diabetes medications (because of cost). Sarah said that she had taken tuberculosis medication while taking diabetes medication and indicated that it was really "hectic" to manage care for both conditions. She also described being shunned by her family when she coughed; her husband, in particular, feared she would infect him with tuberculosis. Sarah also described feeling discriminated against because of her diabetes during family gatherings because she did not eat certain foods. She grieved that people would think she was not eating because the food was not well prepared or because she wanted to show off her wealth by eating only small portions. When Edna inquired about that, Sarah said that diabetes is associated with the wealthy, so people thought she was trying to imitate the rich by following the diabetes diet.

Sarah also described how people perceived HIV to be better than diabetes because HIV can be treated with free medications and people can get well and look "normal." By contrast, patients with diabetes must purchase their own medications and suffer pains more serious than those caused by HIV. Another woman explained that she experienced some weight loss and became frightened; when she told her boyfriend that she needed to go to the hospital, "he blamed me for infidelity." She said, "He told me that the symptoms that I had were HIV related." As a result, she explained, "One day, I decided to go for an HIV test . . . [and] I was HIV negative. I was then diagnosed with diabetes after other tests were done. When I told him about it, he was not convinced about my diabetes; he just believed that I had HIV."

Aid, Treatment, and Inequality

This final section addresses the complexities of treatment that seem to define a central issue of the diabetes-HIV-poverty nexus, as described by one woman with diabetes: "I think people who have HIV are better than [people with] diabetes. This disease has really disturbed me." Even Esther (from the introduction), who had both conditions, focused on how diabetes treatment was difficult to acquire whereas HIV treatment was free. Across our one hundred interlocutors in Kenya, most people focused on how expensive medications for diabetes were, a finding that set diabetes apart from other common conditions, including both HIV and tuberculosis. This was stated explicitly, for example by a participant who stated: "The advantage with HIV is that the ARVs are available, but for diabetes, sometimes it is hard to get medications when one has no money to buy the drugs." Another man emphasized his frustration with the cost of unaffordable medicine: "There are times I'm doing well but there are times that I don't have, you know, the money to go buy drugs with. It is a problem sometimes, and when you go there, you can't just go to the window with a card and say 'I want these drugs.'"

The availability and accessibility of treatments played a powerful role in how people perceived their illnesses. For instance, Kandace described how having tuberculosis was largely a non-issue for her. This is surprising, as tuberculosis remains common among people residing in low-income communities in Nairobi, and it continues to cause a great deal of suffering and death.[26] However, this also demonstrates how tuberculosis control programs have been successful in both education and treatment of the disease—a coup for global health (even despite the scourge of resistant strains), because tuberculosis is a major killer among people with and without HIV. Yet, the introduction of diabetes into such contexts poses an unexpected threat. This threat is linked not only to poverty but also to homes, such as Kandace's shack in Kibera, that are perfect harbors for *Mycobacterium tuberculosis* and in which tuberculosis can easily be transmitted from one person to the other. Diabetes increases the risk for active tuberculosis to take hold in the body threefold, and it increases four times the potential of relapse after tuberculosis treatment.[27] Nevertheless, Kandace's brief comment on tuberculosis underscores how accessibility to treatment for tuberculosis framed the disease as treatable, a non-issue.

The complexities surrounding access to treatment for tuberculosis and HIV and the complete lack of access to affordable diabetes testing and treatment pose not only social and logistical challenges but also ethical ones. Social challenges were exemplified by people like Kandace and

Esther, who described how diabetes served to cover the social stigma associated with HIV, much like it did in Soweto. This social interaction may affect the poverty-diabetes nexus in that the social stigma linked with HIV serves not only as a barrier to diabetes treatment but also as a conduit of shame, stress, worry, and psychological distress. The barrier of stigma, then, only compounds the financial barrier already linked to diabetes. Moreover, the amplification of diabetes-HIV experiences was evident in Esther's story, as HIV moved beyond her social life and into her corporeal experience when she was herself infected. Esther exemplifies how the risk for diabetes among people with HIV cannot be dissociated from the extraordinary success of ARTs that prolong their lives and produce the potential for syndemic interaction in the first place. For instance, one interlocutor made this link clear: "I think the [ARV] drugs when taken for a long time may contribute to diabetes." Such perception (which has been demonstrated in the biomedical literature, too)[28] creates another stigma-generating link between the conditions. Such interactions of the social, political, and corporeal drive the challenges people with diabetes confront in the context of AIDS.

The logistical challenges posed by diabetes are different in Kenya and in South Africa due to their disparate health systems. In Soweto, people grieved about systemic barriers, poor patient-provider interactions, and treatment shopping, and they often gave up dealing with the system altogether.[29] In Nairobi, however, the barriers were even more severe due to the fact that diabetes testing and treatments were dependent on user fees. User fees in Kenya and throughout sub-Saharan Africa have been the focus of extensive scholarly discussion, and the removal of user fees has become a political priority in the past two decades.[30] In 2004, Kenya introduced a uniform reduction of fees for many groups who would essentially then be exempt from paying for medical care; however, because user fees are fundamental to the cash income of health facilities to cover basic operating costs, many facilities continue to require user fees.[31] This is despite the fact that the World Health Organization prioritizes the reduction of user fees for universal health coverage and the powerful evidence that user fees are prohibitive to poor people seeking medical care and can be catastrophic among poor households.[32] The evidence collected from this study illustrates that user fees are prohibitive for people seeking diabetes care, and that the scale of what one must pay excludes many low-income patients from seeking diabetes care in the first place (at least, until they become very sick).

Why Health Financing Matters

This chapter brings to light the role of the health system as an important contributor to diabetes syndemics. Whereas syndemic theory focuses on the vulnerability of a population as the driving force behind the clustering of diseases, recognizing the central role of health financing in driving people toward or away from clinical care is imperative. The data collected for this study show how people (especially women) put their families first; this creates an even greater gender barrier in care-seeking because women tend to prioritize their family's needs before their own. As a result, mothers and grandmothers will often delay seeking medical care until they become very sick, or they will prioritize one disease over another based on what medications are provided without cost. Prioritizing one disease (such as HIV or tuberculosis) and marginalizing another (such as diabetes) not only puts people's overall health at risk but also further complicates syndemic interactions. This is exemplified by the case of Esther, who took her ART while delaying diabetes care; in this case, it might be her ART that created her potential to develop diabetes in the first place. Understanding these unique social-biological and social-psychological interactions that underlie syndemic suffering provides unique insight into the challenges faced by individuals and populations confronting the unequal burden of affliction.

Conclusion

In the introduction, I argued that stories like Esther's elucidate the social pathways that become transduced into diabetes via intrinsic links between hunger and crisis, structural violence and fear, and cumulative trauma and psychiatric distress. Subsequent chapters have recounted stories of women who struggle with diabetes amid convergent social stress, financial insecurities, traumatic memories, chronic and unrecognized emotional pain, and in some cases infection. The book has been organized around two major focal points—the material and the subjective—which illustrate how diabetes is organized within and across societies and how it becomes embodied in individual narratives. These multiple levels of suffering are woven together through syndemic theory, because diabetes clusters closely with other conditions, interacts with these and other social problems, and is driven by social and financial insecurities that materialize in people's chronic illnesses.

Along the way, I have suggested that it is impossible to understand diabetes without recognizing how the condition becomes embodied from place to place. I have presented findings from four contexts as well as the results of many other studies to show how diabetes manifests in different ways biologically and socially across contexts. I found that psychosocial distress is a constant bedfellow to diabetes among my interlocutors, and this is exacerbated by persistent financial insecurities in people's lives. I have argued that diabetes functions in a more pervasive way among individuals who have faced extraordinary social and psychological suffering. In this way, the effects of a lifetime of compounded traumatic and stressful experiences build up and become expressed not only in chronic, untreated psychiatric distress but also metabolically in insulin resistance. Hypervigilance out of fear, anxiety out of uncertainty, and deep emotional pain out of traumatic memories also become entwined in the diabetes experience. The recognized emergence of diabetes among the communities most afflicted by HIV fundamentally transforms the diabetes experience as well, creating new sources of risk and new challenges to compliance and adherence to biomedical narratives.

In Chicago, we visited Beatriz's story to unpack the complicated and undergirding ways in which structural violence, immigration, depression, diabetes, and interpersonal abuse twist together to cultivate poor health in a low-income Mexican immigrant woman. Stories like Beatriz's cannot be dissociated from the politics of immigration, which cultivates a culture of fear and forces people to take any risk to cross dangerous borders for the sake of an uncertain financial and personal future. With families on both sides of the border and dominant narratives about economic prosperity in the United States, many take calculated risks to attain the promise of a brighter future. Women's bodies and minds in many cases become entrapped, as they plant hidden memories of trauma, stuff their emotions with sugary foods and drinks, and yearn for socio-emotional integration with their peers. Diabetes—at least among the women I interviewed in Chicago—cannot be divorced from the complex, localized ways in which the condition becomes embodied and embedded in these women's everyday lives.

In Delhi, we visited Meena's story to think through the complexities that emerge in a context where so many people have diabetes, although among low-income people it is relatively new (or recently detected). The financial insecurities Meena faced were a constant cause of worry, but so were the expectations of achieving material success and living the good life. Intergenerational dynamics, especially between mothers-in-law and daughters-in-law, in some cases created deep anxieties whereas in others created the sense of safety and security through which women navigated their chronic illnesses. Many women's relationships and perceptions of what was good and what was hard changed through their lives. Perhaps the most important finding was that, when compared to relatively wealthier interlocutors, lowest-income people like Meena faced more cumulative stress, chronic and untreated distress, and delayed care-seeking. This is a product of financial insecurity and of the self-sacrifice of caregiving and putting others before one's own physical and mental well-being.

In Soweto, Sibongile provided a new narrative of diabetes that carried with it the social and psychological impact of the HIV and AIDS epidemic. Not unlike the devastating legacy of apartheid and AIDS, diabetes follows the fault lines of social inequality. This has produced an affliction of diabetes that travels the same path followed by experiences of cumulative stress and distress and convergent conditions like HIV and tuberculosis. The relationship between diabetes and HIV is as social as it is biological. Biologically, living on ART creates the opportunity for diabetes to arise, as people now live more than a decade longer with the infection than they would without medications. Socially, those who care for the children orphaned by the AIDS epidemic will continue to displace their own needs—now dictated by chronic illness—due to the epidemic's noxious targeting of healthy and productive individuals who leave behind children for grandparents to raise. The social bind between diabetes and HIV is further complicated by the conflation of routine diabetes care with routine HIV care, cultivating a nefarious stigma that complicates how people think and talk about diabetes. This social stigma may be one of the greatest challenges facing diabetes education, awareness, and care among my interlocutors in the coming decade.

In Nairobi, a similar narrative emerged, although Kandace's experience unveiled how the health system can functionally displace knowledge, care-seeking, and health among some and not others. In this case, the cost of diabetes testing and medications exceeded the possibilities of many individuals and families, causing them to delay care, skip medications, and prioritize other conditions that made better financial sense. This case exemplifies how international donors that set agendas for caring for some diseases (HIV) and not others (diabetes) can have major consequences for people's lives. These funding inequalities are regressive and will continue to impede comprehensive primary care until governments and donors refocus on what fosters good health and invest in a comprehensive reform of national health systems.[1] Moreover, diabetes serves as a looming economic, social, medical, and health threat that in the coming decades may cripple not only health systems but also societies more broadly if not taken seriously (not unlike an emergent infection).[2]

Yet, diabetes differs in meaningful ways across contexts, and many structural and social problems drive the experience of it. The most impactful factor is personal insecurity in both the domestic and public sphere that derives not only from severe and repeated social traumas but also from crippling financial anxieties that produced a constant level of uncertainty. It is undeniable that such constant and extreme suffering gets under the skin; however, recognizing how the narratives diverged across localities provided critical insights into the ways in which diabetes becomes an entirely different illness based on context. For instance, the social stigma linking diabetes to HIV in South Africa and Kenya had a bigger impact on how people cared for their diabetes than any biological interaction between the two conditions. Similarly, the cultural process of normalizing diabetes in Delhi cultivated a form of fatalism that could cause people to delay or overlook self-care more than in other contexts. The political implications of immigration in the United States have had a profound impact on Mexican immigrant women's stress, personal security, and embodied suffering (revealed in part in their diabetes and depression). Finally, the systematic exclusion of some citizens from essential services in Kenya, where those with HIV are more cared for by the state than those with diabetes, fuels the decade-long debate about how regressive user fees can be and how they continue to make people sicker. In this case, global health policy makers who deem some diseases (HIV) worthy and others (diabetes) unworthy of care cultivate an extraordinarily uneven system of deservingness. However, the problem of an unequal health-care system is not exclusive to nations that depend on international aid. Even in wealthy nations such as the United States, where an extraordinary amount of money is spent on health care due to an unregulated market, treatment remains out of reach for many who do not have medical insurance.[3]

In what follows, I propose five ways in which anthropologists, clinicians, and public health practitioners should rethink diabetes. First, I argue that diabetes must be understood largely as a disease of poverty rather than a disease of modernization, a term that has long been associated with the metabolic condition. Second, I argue that diabetes is always syndemic among the socially and economically vulnerable. Third, diagnosis is perhaps the most influential feature of syndemic suffering, which reveals how diabetes itself is experienced completely differently in the body pre- and post-diagnosis. Fourth, diabetes presents as a different condition across sociocultural contexts because it has a social life that fundamentally transforms how the illness is perceived and experienced. Finally, thinking syndemically requires social policies and clinical contexts to be addressed in tandem. I conclude by offering some promising examples that attend to these macro and micro levels of intervention.

Diabetes Is a Disease of Poverty

Rethinking diabetes requires that we recognize that diabetes is primarily and increasingly a disease of poverty. The idea that diabetes is primarily a product of modernization, as Barry Popkin[4] has argued, is based on the fact that in parallel with economic development, increases in Western diets rich in sugars and fats and reduced movement have transformed people's bodies and driven up weight and propensity for diabetes. Thinking about the rise in obesity and diabetes through the prism of the West, however, undermines the fundamentally local ways in which culture and inequality drive the diabetes experience. I argue that it is no longer useful to think about diabetes as a product of modernization because of the diversity of ways in which diabetes manifests biologically, socially, and culturally. Biologically, diabetes risk differs across contexts; this is exemplified by the fact that populations in Asia and sub-Saharan Africa tend to develop diabetes at a younger age and lower body weight than those in Western contexts, which have been more heavily researched. Socially, gender and age shift how people negotiate chronic illness in their lives; women's experiences, for example, diverge significantly from men's due to social obligations such as caregiving and other forms of personal sacrifice. Themes emerging throughout the interviews, such as the need to

divert money for transport to a clinical appointment to meet more immediate needs of family members, reveal how women's sacrifices cannot
be dissociated from their diabetes. Culturally, the foods people eat and
the cultural moment in which diabetes has arisen influence how the condition is refashioned from one context to the next. This is exemplified by
the diversity of foods that drive obesity in different contexts and the varied ways in which healthy food is perceived and consumed within and
across countries.[5] It is also clearly demonstrated in how culture fosters or
stymies stigma. Thus, thinking about diabetes through a theory of modernization creates a global narrative of diabetes emergence. This is mis-
leading, given that local drivers and experiences transform diabetes in
meaningful ways.

Moreover, to the extent that diabetes has shifted from the affluent to
lower-income individuals, it cannot be dissociated from the structural and
social factors that precipitated it. It was not only the opening of markets
to oily, salty, and sweet foods and drinks that posed a risk to lower-income
people; rather, it was the predatory behaviors of corporations that seek
consumers who crave sugar at a low price.[6] Yet this is not a new story.
The anthropologist Sidney Mintz (1985) argued in his iconic book, *Sweetness and Power*, that the onus of sugar in the globalized world is on the
shoulders of consumers as opposed to producers, because the insatiability
for sugar motivates exploitative production. As consumer drive for sugar
consumption grows and expands among low-income populations, sugar
as a cultural or status symbol shifts in relation to the consumer. Mintz
argues that once the lower classes began to consume sugar, as occurred
in England, the commodity lost its position as a status symbol among the
wealthy: "As sugar became cheaper and more plentiful, its potency as a
symbol of power declined while its potency as a source of profit gradually
increased" (1985, 95); the market potential of sugar has expanded globally as the poor have increased sugar consumption.[7] This is personified
in the narratives in this book that show that diabetes cannot be divorced
from the biopolitics of Big Food[8] that makes it difficult to acquire enough
nutrient-rich food and avoid sugars.[9]

This narrative of Big Food also cannot be dissociated from the "geographies of food retail" that structure what foods people eat and where.[10]
These cheap accessible calories have worked their way into evolving life-
scapes defined by changing family dynamics, social roles, and financial

demands within the city—as well as in rural areas, which are not the focus of this book and demand critical study with uniquely different challenges. Raj Patel describes this exploitive syndemic in *Stuffed and Starved*:

> Unless you're a corporate food executive, the food system isn't working for you. Around the world, farmers and farmworkers are dying, with the connivance of elected officials, and at the whim of the market. Through processed food, consumers are engorged and intoxicated. The agribusiness's food and marketing have contributed to record levels of diet-related disease, harming us today and planting a time-bomb in the bodies of children around the world. Supermarket shelves offer an abundance of cheap calories, even as they bleed local economies. We are increasingly disconnected both from production of our food and from the joy of eating it. Most of this happens with consumers ignorant to the suffering that precedes every mouthful of food. And the architecture of our neighbourhoods and working lives makes it impossible to imagine anything better. (2012, 299)

Understanding how structural violence and poverty fundamentally transform diabetes risk in such contexts reveals not only geographic vulnerabilities but also how intertwined food, finances, stress, family, and ecological livelihoods have become.

Further, diabetes emerges along fault lines of social inequality that cannot be dissociated from structural racism and residential segregation that siphon some people into slums and others into wealthy enclaves. These structural undercurrents are as closely linked to diabetes as they are to the unequal afflictions of HIV and tuberculosis. They are also intimately linked to public and private experiences of violence, especially among women, that produce a disproportionate amount of stress; the unity of such violence (sexual, physical, verbal, emotional) across contexts cannot be dissociated from the elevated levels of psychological suffering, gendered subjugation, and embodiment of stress revealed by the women in this book. As diabetes increases among socially and economically disadvantaged populations around the world, the systematic exclusion from affordable healthcare for non-infectious conditions like diabetes becomes more visible. This exclusion is further perpetuated by the way health care is structured, financed, and distributed, especially in health systems that require profits to function.

Diabetes Is Always Syndemic

Rethinking diabetes requires that we understand that diabetes is *always* syndemic among the socially and economically vulnerable. This is in part because poverty and structural violence drive the onset, distribution, and clustering of diabetes and its complications. Recognizing the impact of social and psychological suffering on diabetes is a question of not only the social realm but also the biological. This puts cortisol and inflammation at the center of the diabetes story, moving it beyond fatty and sugary foods and the ways and intensities in which we exercise our bodies. In this way, social pathways are literally transduced into metabolic disease. For instance, based on the ethnographic narrative evidence in this book, we might consider personal insecurities linked to violence in the private and public spaces to be implicit syndemic cofactors to diabetes and depression. At the same time, we must critically interpret the local ways in which the black box of stress diverges from one place to the next. This stress may be communicated using local idioms, somatic symptoms, and even other diseases. Such stress may also mediate how risk for diabetes is conceived and how adherence to diabetes care is construed. Such understanding is imperative when thinking about what clinical interventions might be more effective in one particular place.

As these conditions move along the fault lines of society and settle among the most geographically vulnerable, thinking about historical and social processes that produce and perpetuate these disease clusters becomes a priority. Residential segregation and structural racism that foster food insecurity among some populations and not others are one example of how geographic vulnerabilities can define diabetes risk. However, such processes are not only structural. Historical trauma connected to political violence and race-based segregation and oppression, as in the case of apartheid in South Africa or Jim Crow in the United States, may influence diabetes affliction within communities affected by these forms of structural violence. These examples show how extreme marginalization can physically siphon people off from certain parts of the city through laws; however, they also have longstanding effects on the body that cannot be dissociated from the higher burden of diabetes-related suffering among those who have experienced historical trauma. This argument is based on a theory of epigenetics proposing that historical trauma and oppression may be passed through generations.[11] According to this hypothesis, historical trauma actually turns on and off certain genes through methylation to change the ways in which our bodies respond to the worlds in which we live. These changes to our biology are then reproduced in our children, linking trauma from the past with our present and future.[12] Thus geographic vulnerabilities may be closely linked to biological histories.

Geographic vulnerabilities are also linked to epidemiological histories that produce different clusters of diseases across contexts and therefore create different realities. The legacies of the HIV and AIDS epidemic exemplify this best, revealing how deeply influential ideas about HIV are today on those who are affected or infected by the epidemic. People saying they have diabetes to disguise an HIV diagnosis, and a flip-flop of that strategy whereby diabetes produces a stigma-by-association with AIDS, exemplify this. Perhaps, however, the rise of the tuberculosis-diabetes syndemic exemplifies this best: Living with diabetes in a poorly ventilated home with a family member who has active tuberculosis increases one's risk to acquire the illness up to three times. This correlation echoes the fear that HIV has rung around the world when the rise of HIV-linked immunosuppression caused a resurgence of tuberculosis. Diabetes, too, has the potential to exacerbate this reemerged infection.

Recognizing how structural and social dynamics interact syndemically with diabetes differently across contexts requires that we again reconsider the global narrative for diabetes treatment. The dominant clinical message prioritizes individual-focused motivations, such as diet, exercise, and medicine adherence, which are inherently limiting because they obscure structural and social forces that affect how people think about and engage in self-care. This does not mean that Metformin or insulin injections cannot work to improve one's insulin resistance, or that Wellbutrin may not work for reducing the burden of depression. Instead, we must recognize how some remedies may deal with the social drivers of these co-occurring conditions that intersect, interact, and are mutually exacerbating. Thus, peer support networks, counseling, food supplementation, economic support, housing programs, community health workers, and other socially driven interventions may be as effective as pharmaceutical ones.[13]

This also demands that we rethink how the notion of epidemic might be replaced with that of syndemic in scholarship on health disparities. This is because rarely does an epidemic work in isolation across a population, especially when it encounters poverty and subjugation. Changing how we think about diseases across populations will enable epidemiologists to determine better how geographic vulnerability produces adverse health outcomes. Geographic vulnerability in this sense would implicate two or more health conditions with poverty, social exclusion, gender-based violence, climate change, displacement to agricultural or industrial wastes, and other forms of social and environmental stress. Addressing these clusters of disadvantage statistically is imperative to help policy makers understand how social and economic inequalities facilitate the clustering of diseases among the poor. Doing so will also address some of the discrepancies in how people perceive, measure, and use the syndemic concept in global health.

Diagnosis Matters

Rethinking diabetes requires that we take seriously how diagnosis fundamentally transforms syndemic diabetes in ways that are completely unrelated to biology. For instance, many go undiagnosed for years, only to find they have diabetes when seeking medical care for an acute problem or some symptom of the condition. Becoming someone diagnosed with diabetes is a period of reckoning in regard to what it means culturally, socially, and personally. Culturally, people negotiate how others perceive diabetes and how living with the condition is understood around them. Socially, people consider how they navigate chronic illness in relation to family, friends, and institutions from which they will seek care. Personally, many go through a process of reconsidering the meaning of life itself. It is through this *social* experience of diabetes that syndemic suffering becomes a vehicle for interpreting how culture and society modify the experience of disease clusters in people's lives.

The role of the diagnosis in what it means to have diabetes brings into focus the central issue of the dichotomy between body and experience. Annemarie Mol and John Law (2004) have addressed this question by suggesting a way out of the dichotomy between *having* and *being* a body.

They argue: "As part of our daily practices, we also do (our) bodies. In practice we enact them" (Mol and Law 2004, 45). This does not dismiss the fact that insulin resistance exists *in* the body (biological-biomedical) or that we *are* living with diabetes (experiential-perceptual). Mol and Law (2004, 47) focus on how "day-to-day handling (or avoiding) hypoglycaemia" requires self-awareness as much as clinical monitoring. In this way, diagnosis does not transform people's biological selves; rather, diagnosis transforms their living narratives so that they become people with diabetes. This requires an identity shift, because although people are associated with a condition that they may well have had for many years, having a diagnosis may increase their interactions with the health system and may require them to take care of their condition. It is not only an identity shift but also a shift in reliance on others and in self-care. *Doing* self-care requires phenomenological awareness as well as navigation through cultural, social, and economic prisms that transform what people know should be done versus what can be done to manage their care. As Mol and Law (2004, 54) argue, the body both *acts* (responds) and *enacts* (produces) a response to the environment in which we live, bringing feelings, foods, and friends to interact with the "diabetes it lives with."

This argument can be understood through a reflection on how gendered experiences fundamentally affect illness experiences. On the one hand, the body *acts* (responds) to the violence that so many women endure through heightened cortisol and inflammation, which can be linked to insulin resistance.[14] The psychophysiological responses to such trauma may be stymied or perpetuated by women's responses to violence—they may for example immigrate away from a perpetrator or internalize negative emotions and socially isolate themselves for years. The body also *enacts* (produces) a response to the environment through the intersectional ways in which women respond to their social world post-diagnosis. Gendered subtleties revealed how women reimagined their selves and their roles as caregivers living with diabetes in ways that differed from men's. Despite knowing that they should care for their diabetes, many women put their money and time into the immediate needs of others (whether or not the problem at hand was a "crisis"). In these ways, family dynamics create unique challenges for care-seeking and self-care that require women to demonstrate incredible strength and often (re)negotiate their power.

It is these competing demands that take precedence and demonstrate how agency can be constrained or amplified. When non-medical problems are prioritized over illness, they reveal how the biomedical concept of risk obfuscates the social pathways that produce disease. When risk is (re)negotiated post-diagnosis in such personal ways, and self-care and care-seeking are shelved in order to care for the ones women love most, then diabetes "control" becomes a product of gendered priorities.

This point makes clear the distinctive meaning of suffering in syndemics. Recognizing the role of such suffering is imperative when thinking syndemically; however, because the body is what is measured in syndemic analyses, there is a focus on determining how two or more diseases emerge, travel together, and interact. This is why one may measure a syndemic simply by biomarkers and economic analysis, which has become increasingly a focus of syndemic analyses in public health. Although theorizing what conditions cluster together by way of literature review and epidemiological analyses produces important insights into which syndemics may appear within a population, it overlooks the embodied suffering that is at the heart of syndemic interactions. Syndemic suffering—a critical study of phenomenology—interrogates how the living narrative responds to illness, disease clusters, and the social world. It is imperative to return to these individual experiences to fully understand how experiential dimensions of the clustering matter in people's lives and materialize in the physical body. This is exemplified by the fact that without an analysis of syndemic suffering, one might miss the substantial impacts, for example, of HIV stigma, caregiving, or user fees on care-seeking and self-care for diabetes in Kenya.

The Social Life of Diabetes

Rethinking diabetes requires that we recognize how diabetes may become a different disorder across contexts. Whereas the similarities of gender, violence, distress, and caregiving are somewhat striking across locations, the differences that emerged between contexts provide important insights into how diabetes is fundamentally shaped by culture and society. This point brings us away from the potential causes—oppression, violence, inequality—of poor health and requires that we focus on phenomenological experience as well. This does not mean that the structural and social drivers of diabetes do not matter; rather, I argue that the subjective matters as much as the material. On the one hand, women across contexts describe that suffering is suffering. What makes diabetes different? They contextualize diabetes within their own lives and within the social realities they navigate as they make decisions about what matters to them at that moment. In this way, diabetes is not only a product of social suffering but also a confluence of competing priorities within the social or medical realms.

Stigma is the starkest example of how the social life of diabetes differs across borders. Think for example of the differences in how people perceived and experienced diabetes in India and the United States. In Delhi, people normalized diabetes and compared it to something as ordinary as the common cold, therefore reducing the shame and stigma attached to it. In contrast, stigma, self-blame, and shame are common sentiments co-constructed by individuals seeking biomedical care in Western contexts, including the United States.[15] Such stigma cannot be dissociated from individualized beliefs about diabetes care, which focus on diet and exercise and place blame for the illness exclusively on the patient (as opposed to structural or social problems). Such beliefs require patients to change their behaviors and adhere to their new identities as chronically ill individuals. In contrast, without prevailing notions of shame and blame, a form of fatalism or apathy may have emerged in Delhi that has caused some disillusionment with clinical expectations. This may be related to the normalization of diabetes specifically or to the more general understanding that diabetes ranks low in the hierarchy of important life challenges (especially when compared to the needs of loved ones).

On the other hand, the catch-all stigma found in sub-Saharan Africa tells another story. When bound to HIV stigma, diabetes becomes all but normalized. Sibongile and Esther exemplify how the diabetes diagnosis creates a form of liminality that, as Victor Turner (1969) described in *The Ritual Process,* displaces sick individuals from society because they are (1) physically ailing and (2) stigmatized due to illness. In these contexts, stigmatization is not simply linked to a new, unknown disorder, but it is rather a long-standing belief linked to what some perceive to be amoral behavior and cultural blame. Structural liminality becomes significant at the family level, where families affected by chronic illnesses (from AIDS to diabetes) become burdened by social stigma, caregiving, and transformation of a productive family member who has taken on a "sick role" (where they may be released from normal household duties and expectations).[16] This is another type of transpersonal suffering whereby the stress of some family members is transferred to the family unit.[17] It also produces a form of social contagion of suspicion where diabetes moves into a new realm of "sickness," melding stigmas not by lessening stigma for people living with HIV but rather by heightening stigma for those suffering from other diagnoses that require lifestyle adjustments. Recognizing how HIV stigma manifests in diseases like diabetes and therefore reconstitutes what is communicable by way of social discourse and cultural notions about sickness and treatment reveals an important way in which the social life of diabetes is locally rooted and culturally produced.[18]

Thus, thinking syndemically about the social life of diabetes requires that we attend to the power of culture and ideology in making diabetes distinct across contexts. This idea builds on what Vinh-Kim Nguyen and Karine Peschard (2003, 459) posed as the "embodiment of social relations" that allows "affliction to be related to prevailing ideologies that inform policy, configurations of social violence, the way misfortune is conceptualized and managed, and how meaning systems influence how individuals interpret their bodily states, seek care, and fashion themselves according to prevailing moral notions." For women, this may imply unpacking how caregiving creates a barrier to addressing chronic illness: In each study site, women perceived their chronic illness to be lower on the list of pressing concerns when compared to the basic needs to clothe, feed, and support their family members—even though they said they would use those funds for diabetes care if their husbands had the condition. This is one example of how cultural notions of gender and subjectivity may produce poorer health among women once they develop diabetes. Moreover, political and clinical ideologies that shape the cost and availability of treatments may determine how some diseases are simply perceived to be more deserving than others—a perception steeped in the prioritization of emergent epidemics that has dominated donor-funded aid. In this way, people-centered perspectives can inform how we understand in what ways social dynamics may make an impact on population health.

Syndemic Interventions Matter

Thinking syndemically requires that we think from policy to practice, drawing from the large body of existing knowledge about how to provide care for the whole person. Social and structural inventions that may be eligible for funding from non-medical sources can make a big impact and must be recognized as fundamental to improving health. However, whereas policy-level interventions might make the biggest impact in the prevention of diabetes, having the potential to tackle the epidemic proportions of the problem, they still cannot exist without concurrent clinical interventions that are integrative, holistic, and person centered. Improving educational opportunities, providing micro-loans or a higher minimum wage for people to pull themselves out of poverty, and revolutionizing housing can make an extraordinary impact on people's financial and emotional lives; however, no upstream intervention will be a silver bullet without concurrent interventions that attend to the mind, body, and social suffering that surround people's everyday lives.

Syndemic thinking is built on the notion that policy-level interventions are as imperative as clinical ones. Therefore, it demands that we look at the problem from all angles, drivers, and potential impacts on human life. Table 4 includes a list of potential interventions that may make a big impact in the lives of people who struggle with insulin resistance and the many convergent conditions that accompany it. I provide this list in order to spark the conversation about what moving factors must be integrated together to tackle diabetes. I am not the first to suggest many of these interventions, nor am I the first to suggest that integration is imperative for caring for people with diabetes. Yet, the triangulation of these multiple levels of intervention is largely excluded from the siloed biomedical and public health dialogue about how to intervene for diabetes. For instance, the *Lancet* Taskforce on NCD and Economics has recently advanced the provocative economic argument that household poverty and user fees can have a formidable power in inhibiting people around the world from overcoming non-communicable diseases.[19] This is an incomplete story because, as I have argued in this book, the social and the biological can be as powerful as the economic. Thus, taking seriously what Arthur Kleinman refers to as "what's at stake" requires that we take seriously the sociopolitical

TABLE 4. Syndemic Interventions

Upstream solutions	Clinical interventions	Community interventions	Downstream solutions
Food policy: Regulating sugars in foods by labeling % of daily amount	**House visits**	**House visits for super utilizers**	Community gardens
School food policy: Advocating for improved school lunch options	**Person-centered medical homes:** Clinical coordination to provide care for all health conditions in one consultation	**Community-based mental health:** Improving access to Spanish-speaking counselors; mental health care at community centers; house calls; and apps for counselors to protect privacy and provide emotional support	**Women's groups:** financial planning and education
Housing policy: Improving access to safe housing, legal counsel	**Integrated medical teams:** Teams that include physicians, mid-level health providers (nurses, technicians), social workers, lawyers, and clinical mangers	**Peer group counseling:** Modeled off of the Alcoholics Anonymous model; meetings in public places with private spaces (YMCA, church); Discussions about stress, food, illness, past experiences	**Medical bankrupty forgiveness:** Removing medical debt in contexts where this exists (United States)
Health care policy: Universal health coverage	**Incentivizing providers** for healthy patients	**Addressing rumor and confusing messaging:** this should be context specific, such as addressing perceived links between HIV and diabetes in South Africa	**Lay leadership:** Providing small grants for community-led projects, such as food access projects and community gardens
Minimum wage policy: Raising minimum wage to a livable and equitable level			
Immigration policy: Work visas for undocumented workers			

contexts and moral predicaments of patients and sufferers by recognizing how diabetes and its partners are locally defined, socially navigated, and renegotiated through interactions with society, politics, and the health system.[20]

Recommendations for Thinking Syndemically Upstream

Address Social Inequality   There are two key policy recommendations to address social inequalities: taxing the wealthy to pay for social programs and raising the minimum wage. On the one hand, an article in the *Lancet* has recently argued that the household level of financial security, including having health insurance or not, maintains a strong connection with improved health among those living with conditions like diabetes.[21] With increasing wealth inequalities throughout the world,[22] failing to tax those with the most wealth prioritizes corporations and elites over the majority of citizens. This taxation should not be a blanket tax. Rather, it should target those who benefit the most from food politics: Big Food industries and medical technology companies driven by profit. Large food corporations benefit an extraordinary amount from people consuming highly caloric and highly processed foods, whereas companies that produce medical products benefits from the biomedical interventions utilized to intervene on them, from bariatric surgery to insulin injections. These companies have no incentives to promote community health and well-being and extensive economic incentives to work against many of the community-based ideas suggested here. A substantive tax for their oversight, however, together with tax breaks for investing in community health, may make the tide turn.

Tax Sugar   Marion Nestle (2013, 2015) has argued powerfully that taxing Big Sugar could ameliorate some of the greatest threats to people's health, modeling this theory after the successful campaigns against Big Tobacco. In an evaluation of waist size and food markets from 173 countries, a group of social epidemiologists led by Sanjay Basu (2012) has argued that sugar is the reason that urbanization and income have become correlated in diabetes rates. They found that income tends to increase in relation to overall food-market size in low- and middle-income countries, but waist size is not exclusively linked to income. In other words, they argue that it is the consumption of sugar that explains the rise in diabetes, and not urbanization or income (which have so commonly been linked to modernization). They argue that the level of food importation significantly shifts the context of global markets, and reveals how sugar and other sweeteners are directly linked to widening waistlines.[23] Returning to Mintz (1985), it is not the fattening of wallets but rather the increase of sugar availability in foods and beverages that explains the rise of diabetes at the country level, especially among lower-income populations who gain easier access to oily, salty, and sweet foods. Even more, the sugar industry has succeeded in obfuscating how much sugar is in foods by removing the percentage of daily sugar in each product (and often replacing it with "fats"), although such measure is included for all other ingredients.[24]

Housing Interventions Are Health Interventions   Thinking about housing as a health intervention for diabetes involves multiple layers of complexity. For instance, some women described how feeling unsafe within their home provoked extraordinary stress, and in some cases profound psychological distress. Many described how feeling unsafe or uncomfortable walking in public spaces impeded their adherence to clinical recommendations to exercise. Others described problems within their home that were structural—such as mold, lack of ventilation, or lack of space. Other housing issues may include law enforcement for domestic violence against children and women. Such issues address factors that go from personal security and stress to respiratory illness, from asthma to tuberculosis. This may be tackled at the policy level, or it may be addressed by providing accessible and free legal counsel inside the medical clinic.

Other health interventions may be as broad and systemic as desegregation, a fundamental move that may increase access to better schools and grocers and improve personal security, especially for elderly community members. Considering desegregation as a health intervention requires a radical rethinking of social policy as health policy. Such thinking expands how we think about health and disease and refocuses our efforts upstream. Although these ideas are not new, a serious consideration of how social determinants such as safe and affordable housing can affect mental and physical health continues to be sidelined. For instance, what would happen if the NIH made such interventions a priority?

Whereas some goals may be achieved only at a higher policy level, others may involve ground-up innovation that may hold the potential for local transformation. For instance, DC Greens, a small food advocacy organization in Washington, DC, piloted a program that promotes access to a variety of fresh vegetables in the widely distributed corner stores in areas commonly deemed to be food deserts. After a pilot project, they found that corner stores continued selling fresh veggies if they were able to stock a fridge full with them and provide consumers with a variety of foods (as opposed to a limited supply). Such an approach points to the need to enhance economic opportunity for local entrepreneurs and the variety of fresh fruits and veggies people can access near their homes.

User Fees Are Regressive   Thinking syndemically requires that we consider how universal health care can transform people's health.[25] The health system shaped the experience of many women in this study by determining how they would access medical care, from whom they would receive it, what medicines would be available and accessible, what technologies would be affordable and available for testing and diagnostics, and how they—poor patients who struggled to put food on the table—would be expected to pay for it. The health systems of the United States, India, South Africa, and Kenya incorporate both private and public funding for medical care, with private health insurance being linked with occupation and public health care programs serving low-income patients. Achieving health equity, and thereby ensuring that patients have accessible and affordable medicines for their complex health conditions, requires efficient and just health systems that can respond to local contexts and needs.[26] Because many health systems are unequal and provide inadequate care for low-income populations, many of the chronically ill with small incomes have difficulty accessing the health system and receiving long-term care. A study from South Africa demonstrated that of those who reported having a chronic condition, half had reported seeking no medical care in the past month and only one-third had received consistent medical care.[27] In some cases, user fees are a major barrier to accessing medicines, routine testing, and other health needs.[28] In other cases, especially when governments provide medical testing and medications free of cost, food and transportation costs to the clinic become "user fees" and reveal the inability of such policies to engage holistically with health building. Thus, barriers to care-seeking extend to the social world, demonstrating how intimately our social lives dovetail our medical lives.

Promote Universal Primary Care   This point brings us back to the long-standing debate in global public health: Should primary health care be comprehensive or selective? After the political allegiance to primary health care in the Alma Ata Declaration in 1978, and the political momentum it generated, the decades that followed illustrated a powerful push in the opposite direction. There are many good examples of progress toward primary health care,[29] and especially the movement for universal health coverage,[30] as well as a recommitment to advancing primary health care for all with the signing of the Astana Declaration in 2018. Yet, the politics and funding priorities of public health interventions undermine the building of health systems, promoting instead selective technocratic interventions that target diseases that are measurable and reportable to those who hold the purse strings.[31] With the Bill and Melinda Gates Foundation holding the reigns of global health in a way that is unprecedented of any private individual or foundation in human history,[32] shifting away from prioritizing technical fixes is unlikely. Yet, political pressure is needed to swing the pendulum back and invest in the primary health care systems necessary to combat the threat of diabetes and other non-communicable diseases. There is no doubt that continuing to focus on vertical programming, which directs money away from investments into health systems and prioritizes diseases at the pleasure of the donors, will continue to stymie real progress in building up healthy populations. Whereas this is true on a global scale, the United States exhibits one of the most notorious examples of politics impeding healthcare for all. Despite improvements associated with the Affordable Care Act, many people remain uninsured with tenable access to healthcare because, even though there is substantial evidence of what we should and could do, there is not enough political will to achieve it. As long as equity is sidelined and profit is prioritized, health in the United States will continue to deteriorate. The stories presented in this book exemplify these truths.

Recommendations for Thinking Syndemically at the Clinical Level

Integrated Clinical Care   People are extremely busy, and simply arriving at the clinic can take extraordinary effort. One of the most relevant findings from the clinical narratives in this book is that clinical care must be more integrated to facilitate people's ability to both understand and care for multiple diagnoses, clinical recommendations, and social pressures. For instance, people must be able to go to the clinic, receive comprehensive medical care for all their conditions, and leave with medications, counseling, and comprehensive care plans that are person focused. More holistically, comprehensive medical care would also incorporate legal services to enable patients to address potential environmental drivers of personal suffering (such as mold-induced asthma). This can be achieved by task-sharing medical care—whereby physicians serve in a supervising role and clinics integrate care by including nurse practitioners, case workers, lawyers, social workers, and psychologists.[33]

One example of this collaboration is a partnership of medical schools in western Kenya, often known as AMPATH, or Academic Model of Providing Access to Healthcare.[34] AMPATH is broadly recognized in global health as an unusually symbiotic partnership between Moi Medical School in Kenya and Indiana University Medical School in the United States (although now there are many more international partners). AMPATH has pioneered some of the most integrated care for HIV by recognizing early on during the epidemic how hunger and poverty affected those seeking HIV care.[35] They argued that hunger and ART produced a synergistic relationship, and therefore created interventions that addressed the synergistic (or syndemic) relationships among poverty, hunger, HIV, and ART. At AMPATH, those who receive HIV services also are evaluated for food and financial security. These programs focus on improving nutrition and reducing hunger among those on ART. They also provide microenterprise and agricultural training to help those in treatment to make ends meet. Now these programs include psychosocial support groups for those who are affected by or infected with HIV; this is in part because social determinants (including gender) are more powerful predictors of depression than serostatus.[36] More recently, they found that hypertension and diabetes couple in those infected with HIV and incorporated screening and treatment into primary care.[37] Unlike most medical programs, AMPATH puts community needs at the center of its work and prides its success on its malleability to the ever-changing AIDS epidemic. Such adaptiveness becomes increasingly pertinent as syndemics emerge and we continue to learn more about what conditions are co-constructed by shared social drivers and biological and biomedical interactions.

Another model for achieving integrated chronic care through an existing HIV/AIDS platform was put forth by Partners in Health for Rwanda's Ministry of Health.[38] This program reveals how chronic care is not only beneficial but also makes the most sense in some of the poorest health systems because it addresses multiple conditions at once. In Rwanda, HIV treatment and psychiatric care were decentralized from large urban hospitals to community-level interventions that relied on community health workers to manage treatment and care of HIV and mental health in rural areas where nearly 80 percent of Rwandans reside. This HIV/AIDS platform was then leveraged for surveillance of and healthcare delivery for noncommunicable diseases like diabetes (for which incidence and prevalence were relatively low). This model worked in Rwanda in part because conditions like diabetes were viewed as carrying a marginal cost compared to the prevailing infectious diseases. Thus, this model exemplifies how screening and management for conditions like diabetes can fit into existing HIV/AIDS platforms when such care is inhibited by cost and lack of human resources. Yet, such a model does not address the potential social stigma associated with linking diabetes to existing HIV/AIDS platforms, or how such models of integration may be relayed to high-density urban settings.

A related idea is team-based care, whereby a team of professionals comanage a panel of patients; an example might be a team of one psychologist, three to six doctors or nurse practitioners, two to three community health workers, and two registered nurses. The physicians would diagnose chronic conditions and treat acute problems, the nurses would provide in-depth chronic disease education, the community health workers would pull on their deep knowledge of the community's lived experience to provide health advice, and the psychologists would attend to psychosocial issues. The team would collectively address the confluence of factors that define a syndemic for a large panel of patients within a targeted geographic area. The workforce and resource requirements for this model are extensive, but it points to opportunities to expand current task-sharing models to include team members not traditionally included, such as mental health workers. In addition, some of these team members may work within the community, visiting homes and bypassing transportation barriers that may prevent some from visiting the clinic.

Clinical Messages Matter   The growing mantra of those fighting the obesity epidemic in the United States and elsewhere emphasizes that exercise will not be enough to overcome the increasing rates of obesity and diabetes. In some cases, advising patients to exercise regularly—although clearly positive for their health—is not only infeasible but also insufficient. On the one hand, routine exercise may be infeasible for many of the issues we have already discussed (such as the lack of a safe and comfortable place to walk); on the other hand, it may not be enough to overcome high-calorie diets. This returns us to the argument that regulating hidden sugar in food and the abundance of quick, cheap, overprocessed foods is a pressing issue. It also puts a spotlight on our need to understand structural competencies[39]—or the need to recognize how a broader array of competing factors influence what people do, how they think, and how these factors influence sickness and health. This involves the need for clinicians and nutritionists to rethink the primary messages they communicate to their patients and to convey messages that resonate with them—for example, modifying diets in meaningful, respectful ways and not necessarily to conform to national standards. Thinking through how individuals can adapt their diets to incorporate healthier foods that do not compete with their preferred ways of eating is fundamental.

Understanding how social and cultural factors may impede people's ability to meet clinical expectations is exemplified by the narratives in this book that emphasize how cultural expectations of sacrifice and caregiving for others run against a focus on personal health concerns. Many women put their family's food preferences before their own dietary needs, preparing, serving, and consuming common foods with their family members. Others hide their visible suffering by refraining from asking family members to help with biomedical tasks, such as picking up medication. These findings reflect Weaver's (2016, 8) research among Northern Indian women, in which many women expressed how they "leave their own care up to God and focus on their families instead."[40] This is another example of the need for structural competency in which gendered subtleties play powerful roles in how people cook, eat, and care for their bodies in ways that compete with clinical recommendations.

Stress, Including Traumatic Stress, Cannot Be Dissociated from Diabetes   Recognizing how closely linked trauma and diabetes are socially, psychologically, and physiologically is fundamental for treating the condition. This requires that counseling for ongoing social stress, emotional distress, traumatic memories, and other convergent emotional suffering be at the center of clinical care for cardio-metabolic conditions like diabetes. Without addressing the emotional issues at the center of people's lives, caring for chronic illness will be difficult as deep-seated emotional histories will continue to perpetuate chronic suffering.

Within the clinic, mental health care must be considered standard of care. Making mental health care integral to diabetes care would be a first step toward improving health among low-income populations.[41] Direct one-on-one counseling must be more available and affordable for people who have experienced severe trauma, extreme poverty, and diabetes complications. Moreover, group psychotherapy interventions hold promise for select populations even in extremely low-resource settings with high burdens of political violence and poverty.[42] Gender-specific support groups must become routine in diabetes care and should be available for all patients, especially for those with poor or worsening diabetes control. Clerks, nursing staff, and physicians should all be required to inform high-risk patients of the services available and to encourage their attendance. This requires team-based medicine that focuses on the most pressing needs and best practices for the most vulnerable patients.

Recommendations for Thinking Syndemically at the Community Level

House Calls Matter   There are a number of examples of programs that make house calls, and most of them serve the poorest people in society. Jeffrey Brenner's work in Camden, New Jersey, on the super utilizer (SU) strategy, for example, is an effective and holistic approach from the United States. Super Utilizers are people who frequent emergency rooms with empty pockets and severely poor health, driving up costs and concerns within the health-care system. In most cases, they delay care-seeking because they have had poor experiences with the health system, are from historically marginalized communities, and/or suffer from co-occurring mental illness and substance abuse. The SU strategy translated the law enforcement strategy of hot spots to medicine, targeting high-risk individuals and communities who frequent emergency rooms. Instead of waiting for these people to come to the health-care system with an emergency, the SU strategy goes to them. Just like law enforcement allocates resources to high-crime areas, hot spots in medicine allocate resources to those who pose high risk of repeated emergency visits.[43] This involves community-based care coordination through a home visit program that connects a SU with primary care and community resources. This is the essence of a clinical redesign whereby those who care for the sickest patients walk with them in their communities and deal with the social determinants that undermine their health. Often these care coordinators are licensed practical nurses, medical assistants, or social workers—those in the medical system who are most accustomed to navigating the US health-care bureaucracies and making sure that social support and health care get to those who need them most. Many have argued that this is not only the most effective way to transform the health of the poorest people in the city, but also the most cost effective.[44] It is also the most dignified way to bring care to those who need it most.

Community-Based Peer Support Feeling heard by others who share the same experiences and thinking through potential solutions with peers can be transformative. This may include speaking, storytelling, writing, and especially connecting with someone who has a shared experience. For others, engaging with someone who cares through an app may be a useful solution. For example, having someone trained in cognitive-based therapies check in daily by text to make sure someone is dealing okay with past emotions, current stressors, or chronic illness management may make a big difference—especially on those days when people need a follow-up or someone to speak with, such as after the loss of a loved one, a financial crisis, or an experience of violence.[45] Not in the least, such support may help people face the loneliness that often accompanies chronic illness, and it should always be available for people living with chronic illness that requires complex care within and apart from a medical setting.

Community support groups, however, are not only for talking about feelings. People also support each other by teaching and learning to inject needles, manage sugar spikes, and organize multiple medications—as well as how to eat better, how to store and utilize medication, and how to decide when medication is imperative and when it is not (especially when people have to strategically choose between their medication and other family basic needs). These are all good examples that illustrate how to weave together care for social, psychological, and physical problems. For instance, recent examples of mental health interventions integrated into maternal and child health services reveal how the strong link between the two domains can actually empower community health workers to make a bigger impact through their work.[46] Other examples may involve community health workers visiting homes in urban slums to help to ensure that patients attend clinic visits, access essential medicines, and manage their multiple morbidities. Thinking syndemically might require community health workers to incorporate a standard checklist of myriad symptoms to evaluate high-priority social and health conditions—from tuberculosis to nutrition, smoking, overcrowded living conditions, and weak social networks. Once the general screening identifies or negates these priority conditions, individuals undergo an extensive evaluation and set up an integrated treatment plan in the primary health center with recognition of the complex social and medical conditions that coexist.[47] The Philips Foundation is currently piloting such programs through Community Life Centers in Kenya.[48] Yet, a major challenge for such an approach is a biomedical bias toward perceiving such care as non-medical; for example, Ippy Kalofonos's (2014) ethnographic work in Mozambique illustrates how people perceive praying as ineffective and outside the purview of clinically oriented work when in fact it may be an essential path for healing.[49]

Chronic Care Can Be Improved through Community Health Workers in All Contexts   A fundamental need for thinking syndemically is task sharing. Task sharing, also called task shifting, is a concept utilized across the health system[50] to indicate tasks often conducted by specialists together with less-skilled health workers who receive specific training for that task.[51] For example, a specialist may be a physician or nurse with specialized training (such as a psychiatrist or psychiatric nurse) and a nonspecialist may be a generalist, from a general practitioner to a nurse or community health worker. Many non-specialists can carry out the detection or distribution of medications; but, more generally, this may be a shift down the chain of command, whereby a specially trained nurse or community health worker can carry out the specific tasks of a more skilled health worker. This shift has the potential to increase access to valuable health resources in places where specialists are not available, but it might also serve well when specialists are available but unwilling or overburdened with responsibilities (such as paperwork and the most severe medical cases). Task sharing should alleviate the burden of the specialists by sharing it with multiple caregivers across the medical system, thereby spreading knowledge about the health care system and increasing access to sufferers who need to be heard and responded to the most.

An important shift for syndemic thinking is that those who task-share should focus on addressing the complexities of whole persons. This requires community health workers to work within a narrower geographic space, where more people are clustered together (especially within hot spots of people disaffected by syndemic problems). By focusing on a smaller radius, community health workers will have more time to recognize the complex and overlapping conditions that encapsulate syndemic problems. This might include less visible responses to social and political determinants of health, such as crippling anxiety, depression, domestic violence, or social isolation. Moreover, working within a smaller geographic area would also enable more community-focused engagements around food, feelings, friends, fears, pains, new conditions, and interactions with the health-care system. The role of the community health care worker, therefore, would be in part that of a cultural broker as well as a trusted source of ongoing guidance and care. It is also important to emphasize that the people in these roles must be paid a fair living wage. Indeed, many community members are not only serving the needs of the broader society, but also, as Esther so clearly conveyed, suffering from the complexities of syndemics, too.

Thinking syndemically requires bringing together the complex ways in which the mind, the body, and sociopolitical dimensions of suffering interact to produce diabetes and its partners from one context to the next. The narratives in this book have illustrated how people around the world experience syndemic diabetes differently, and how important it is to take seriously the cultural, social, and political factors that transform illness experiences. These three levels of intervention will differ from place to place—depending on what local needs are most pressing and what political interventions are most possible at a particular time. In many ways, macro-level interventions—albeit the most transformative at the population level—are the most difficult to implement without political will (which is especially difficult to generate when profits are put first). Micro-level interventions create possibilities for people to cope with illness through integrated care and to build community to cultivate a better future, despite the extraordinary challenges—including diabetes—that so many people face. Building on people's ingenuities and commitments to families and communities will be a source of untangling trauma from the mind and the body to produce better health for people everywhere.

NOTES

Foreword

1. See Nichter 2001.

2. Labeling diabetes as epidemic entails a sematic expansion of the use of the term "epidemic" from denoting infectious disease to indicating disease that affects a large number of people, with a recent and substantial increase in the number of cases (Rosenberg 1992). Connotations of the term "epidemic," what it indexes when applied to NCDs, and how this influences individual and institutional responses in different cultures require close examination (Seeberg and Meinert 2015).

3. See Zimmet 2017.

4. Research has found that undernutrition predisposes children in developing countries to malnutrition-modulated diabetes mellitus (MMDM) later in life, whereas psychosocial stress leads to metabolic dysregulation, a flattening of the normal diurnal cortisol curve, disturbed sleep, impaired glucose regulation, insulin resistance, and arterial inflammation.

5. See the following articles on the convergence of communicable and noncommunicable diseases: Bygbjerg 2012; Frenk and Gómez-Dantés 2017; Oni and Unwin 2015; Remais et al. 2013.

6. See Casqueiro, Casqueiro, and Alves 2012.

7. See Mendenhall 2015a, 2017; Weaver and Mendenhall 2014.

8. See Finkler 2000.

Introduction

1. Throughout the book, I use "HIV," "AIDS," and "HIV and AIDS" to mean different things, in accordance to the use made by other scholars in public health. I use "HIV" alone to represent the experience of living with the virus—often on ART—before someone becomes very sick. I use "HIV and AIDS" to represent the cumulative experience of one's life with the illness and/or a collection of experiences of various people through time (those with HIV and those with AIDS). I do not use "AIDS" alone because few people I interacted with were dying from the condition; however, sometimes I refer to the "AIDS epidemic" to refer to the complete experience of the epidemic.

2. The 2015 *IDF Diabetes Atlas* reports that in 2015, 269.7 million people in urban areas and 145.1 million people in rural areas had diabetes. These numbers are expected to rise to 477.9 million people in urban areas and 163.9 million people in rural areas by 2040, illustrating a rapid rise in diabetes in less than three decades. Of all the individuals with diabetes, 80 percent reside in the Global South (IDF 2015).

3. See Mintz 1985. Marion Nestle (2013, 2015) has carried out some of the most significant pioneering work on nutrition and corporate interests; see also Patel 2012; Stuckler and Nestle 2012; Taubes 2011, 2017.

4. See Lieberman 2003; McGarvey 2009; McGarvey et al. 1989. See also these key papers from nutritional epidemiology: Popkin 2006, 2015; Popkin, Adair, and Ng 2012; Popkin and Hawkes 2015.

5. As opposed to type 1 diabetes (which is congenital and in which children cannot produce insulin) and gestational diabetes (which in many cases goes away after the mother recovers from pregnancy, delivery, and associated challenges), type 2 diabetes develops through a slow process of worsening insulin resistance; however, type 2 diabetes can in some cases be reversed, with insulin levels stabilizing to normal levels.

6. See Lieberman 2003, 2008.

7. See Ahlqvist et al. 2018.

8. See Solomon 2016; Yates-Doerr 2015.

9. See Agardh et al. 2011.

10. See IDF 2015.

11. See Lang and Heasman 2015; Patel 2012; Stuckler and Nestle 2012.

12. See, among others, Ferzacca 2012; Mendenhall 2012; Mendenhall et al. 2010; Rock 2003; Scheder 1988.

13. See Ferreira and Lang 2006.

14. See Narayan et al. 2011.

15. See Carruth and Mendenhall 2018; Smith-Morris 2008.

16. See IDF 2015.

17. See the significant work on epigenetics of metabolic disease: Kuzawa and Sweet 2009; Thayer and Kuzawa 2011; Thayer and Non 2015. On the psychophysiology of stress and diabetes, see Daniel et al. 1999; Golden et al. 2007; Lovallo and Thomas 2000; Pouwer, Kupper, and Adriaanse 2010; Sapolsky 2004.

18. See Ferzacca 2000.

19. See McDade et al. 2006; Thayer et al. 2016.

20. See Berkman et al. 2000.

21. See Weaver 2016.

22. See Bor et al. 2013.

23. See Ludwig et al. 2011.

24. See McEwen and Seeman 1999.

25. See Marmot 2007.

26. See some of the most significant anthropological scholarship on diabetes and social suffering in North America: Ferreira and Lang 2006; Ferzacca 2000, 2012; Hunt, Valenzuela, and Pugh 1998; Mendenhall et al. 2010; Montoya 2011; Rock 2003; Scheder 1988; Schoenberg et al. 2005; Smith-Morris 2008.

27. See Mendenhall 2012.

28. See Mendenhall et al. 2010, which underscores the role of diabetes as an idiom of distress among Mexican immigrant women.

29. At the time it was estimated to be the most populous diabetic population globally; however, now it is considered second to China, followed by the United States.

30. My team interviewed people who resided together in the same region of the city and shared the same religion (Hinduism), making the neighborhood characterization a key difference between them. Although everyone spoke Hindi, regional differences in origin, as most people in Delhi have migrated from somewhere, persisted.

31. The International Diabetes Federation regularly publishes updates to the *Diabetes Atlas*, providing estimates of diabetes prevalence over time and projections. Guariguata and colleagues (2014) published a recent estimate according to which South Africa hosted the most people living with diagnosed and undiagnosed diabetes in sub-Saharan Africa (around 9 percent).

32. See Mendenhall 2015b; Mendenhall and Norris 2015.

33. See Basso 1996; Behar 2003; Farmer 2001; Kleinman 1980, 1988; Mattingly 1998; Menary 2008; Radin 1983.

34. Here are some of the most impactful anthropological perspectives on narrative and chronic illness: Garro 2000; Hunt 1998; Hunt, Browner, and Jordan 1990; Mattingly and Garro 2000; Smith-Morris 2008, 2010.

35. See Bernard 2006. I was also fortunate to attend the National Science Foundation's Summer Institute for Research Design led by Russ Bernard, Susan Weller, and Jeff Johnson, which made a considerable impact on how I think about methods and on the methods I selected for the research presented in this book.

36. Learn more about the CARRS Cohort Study here: http://diabetes.emory.edu/research/CARRS-Cohort.html.

37. Learn more about the Birth to Twenty Plus Cohort here: https://www.wits.ac.za/health/research-entities/birth-to 20/birth-to-twenty/.

38. Learn more about the Africa Mental Health Foundation, the organization with whom I partnered in Nairobi, Kenya, here: http://www.africamentalhealthfoundation.org/.

39. The multiple articles associated with this larger body of work are listed in the bibliography.

40. See Schulz and Mullings 2006, a foundational work on intersectionalities that shaped my thinking about how intersections of gender, sexuality, race, and class affect how people describe a life; interact with diabetes, mental illness, and health care; and situate their experiences within broader political-economic and social frameworks.

1. Syndemic Diabetes

1. See the *Lancet* Series on Syndemics published on March 2, 2017 (Mendenhall 2017; Mendenhall et al. 2017; Singer et al. 2017; Tsai et al. 2017; Willen et al. 2017).

2. This is directly from the *Lancet* Series on Depression and Diabetes (Snoek, Bremmer, and Hermanns 2015, 452).

3. See multiple studies, reviews, and comments on how diabetes emerges and clusters with depression among low-income communities: Agardh et al. 2011; Leone et al. 2012; Mezuk et al. 2013; Pouwer, Kupper, and Adriaanse 2010; Talbot and Nouwen 2000.

4. A growing body of research, including multiple systematic reviews, argues for the bi-directionality of depression and diabetes; see for example Holt, De Groot, and Golden 2014; Renn, Feliciano, and Segal 2011.

5. Structural violence has become a fundamental tenet of medical anthropology and of our understanding of the historical motivations of health inequalities. Some of the earliest work conducted by Johan Galtung in the field of peace studies (see Galtung 1969) provides the theoretical foundation for the theory, but Paul Farmer has famously moved the concept forward within critical medical anthropology through his famous work in Haiti, the United States, Rwanda, Russia, and elsewhere. See for example Farmer 1996, 1997a, 1997b; Farmer, Lindenbaum, and Delvecchio Good 1993.

6. See Farmer 2001; Farmer et al. 2013.

7. See Willen 2007.

8. See Willen 2007, 13.

9. See Bourgois 2001, 2009; Scheper-Hughes 1992.

10. On its website, the Mayo clinic lists type 2 diabetes risk factors to be exclusively weight, inactivity, family history, race, age, gestational diabetes, polycystic ovary syndrome, high blood pressure, and abnormal cholesterol and triglyceride levels. The definitions of these risk factors are circumspect; for instance, the explanation of "race" is, "Although it's unclear why, people of certain races—including blacks, Hispanics, American Indians, and Asian-Americans—are at higher risk." See http://www.mayoclinic.org/diseases-conditions/diabetes/basics/risk-factors/con-20033091.

11. Beagley and colleagues found that globally an estimated 45.8 percent, or 174.8 million, of all diabetes cases in adults are undiagnosed, ranging from 24.1 percent to 75.1 percent across data regions. An estimated 83.8 percent of all cases of undiagnosed diabetes mellitus (type 2) are in low- and middle-income countries. At the country level, Pacific Island nations have the highest prevalence of undiagnosed people with diabetes (Beagley et al. 2013).

12. See Schneider and Moore 2000.

13. According to Sapolsky (2004), when humans experience acute stressors, the sympathetic nervous system projects a response to the body, mediating the four F's: flight, fight, fright, and sex. In such a response, vital hormones, epinephrine and norepinephrine, are released into the general circulation, and the activity of enzymes that regulate catecholamines biosynthesis is stimulated. Through these pathways, the mind instigates a bodily response within seconds. Another key interrelationship between the mind and the body in the stress response is the function of the hypothalamus, which secretes an array of releasing hormones into the hypothalamic-pituitary circulatory system that contribute to the release of CRH (corticotropin releasing hormone), which triggers the pituitary to release the hormone ACTH (corticotropin), which triggers the adrenal gland to release glucocorticoid (a hormone that functions similarly to epinephrine but is released over a matter of minutes or hours, rather than seconds). Together, glucocorticoids, epinephrine, and norepinephrine account for the majority of the immediate psychophysiological responses to stress.

14. Chronic exposure to interpersonal violence may drive hypothalamic-pituitary-adrenal axis processes that alter metabolism, food preferences, and protection from disease (Lee, Tsenkova, and Carr 2012). Several studies have demonstrated that ACEs increase risk for physical and mental health disorders (Danese et al. 2009; Felitti et al. 1998). Differential clustering of risk factors, from local food practices to exposure to violence, combined with variation in access to risk reduction and protective measures will contribute to the emergence of different syndemics across settings.

15. The Centers for Disease Control and Prevention provide a list of articles from the ACE studies by topic area on their website: https://www.cdc.gov/violenceprevention/acestudy/journal.html. The following articles focused on depressive symptoms, obesity, and

heart failure are the most relevant to this study: Chapman et al. 2004; Dong et al. 2004a, 2004b; Edwards et al. 2003; Felitti et al. 1998).

16. Researchers have identified psychophysiological mechanisms linking severe traumas and post-traumatic stress disorder (PTSD), depression, and diabetes (Daniel et al. 1999; Epel et al. 2000, 2001; Fuchsberger et al. 2016; Gunnnar 2000; Kadam et al. 2014; Kessler and Bromet 2013; Kessler et al. 2009; Kuzawa and Sweet 2009; Lee, Tsenkova, and Carr 2012; Ludwig et al. 2011; McEwen and Seeman 1999; Pouwer, Kupper, and Adriaanse 2010; Prince et al. 2007; Thayer and Kuzawa 2011).

17. Moulton, Pickup, and Ismail 2015. These interconnections are outlined extensively in the growing literature on the psychophysiology of diabetes and depression (Talbot and Nouwen 2000; Musselman et al. 2003; Knol et al. 2006; Golden et al. 2007, 2008; Holt, de Groot, Golden 2014; Petrak et al. 2015).

18. See Epel et al. 2000; Wynne et al. 2005.

19. See Wynne et al. 2005.

20. See Kirmayer, Lemelson, and Barad 2007.

21. See Epel et al. 2001.

22. See Pouwer, Kupper, and Adriaanse 2010, as well as other work by Frans Pouwer.

23. See International Society for Developmental Origins of Health and Disease, at https·// dohadsoc.org/.

24. Refer to studies by David Barker (Barker 1995, 1999; Barker et al. 1989).

25. There are three key physiological facts behind the developmental origins hypothesis. First, individuals who are born small have reduced muscle mass, which reduces their energetic requirements. This fact is important because the amount of muscle that an individual has largely determines the amount of energy used during activity or while at rest. Second, low—birth weight babies have greater energetic storage per unit of body mass, which results in greater fat mass. Third, abdominal fat cells are more sensitive to hormonal signals that cause release of fats into the bloodstream among individuals who are born small, resulting in easier access to fat stores during caloric shortfalls (see Baker et al. 2008; Ewald 2008; adapted from Kuzawa 2008).

26. Refer to the following studies in Trevathan, Smith, and McKenna 2008: Baker et al. 2008; Ewald 2008; Kuzawa 2008; Lieberman 2008

27. See Kuzawa and Quinn 2009.

28. See Kuzawa 2008; Kuzawa and Sweet 2009; Thayer and Kuzawa 2011.

29. Research by Chris Kuzawa, Elizabeth Sweet, and Zaneta Thayer illuminates that epigenetics is intergenerational (Kuzawa 2008; Kuzawa and Sweet 2009; Thayer and Kuzawa 2011).

30. See the DOHAD study by Norris et al. 2012.

31. See Fuchsberger et al. 2016.

32. See Rich 2016.

33. Refer to these key Whitehall Studies: Marmot and McDowall 1986; Marmot et al. 1978; Rose 1981, 1985. See also these key social determinants of health studies: Marmot 2005, 2007; Stringhini et al. 2017.

34. See also Krieger 1994, 2001; Krieger and Davey Smith 2004.

35. The three attributes of syndemics are described throughout Merrill Singer's impressive work (Singer 1994, 1996, 2009; Singer and Clair 2003; Singer et al. 2000, 2017).

36. See Zabetian et al. 2014. This is not to dismiss the increasing diffusion of diabetes in rural areas, as the escalation of obesity and diabetes in such areas is evident on a global scale.

37. This table was developed by my student H. Stowe McMurry, now in medical school. Stowe found and/or confirmed many of these statistics; this table was also used in Mendenhall et al. 2017.

38. The data were pulled from the following epidemiological studies: American Diabetes Association 2014; Ayah et al. 2013; CBHSQ 2015; CDC 2015; Claassens et al. 2014; Crowther and Norris 2012; Denning and DiNenno 2010; Guariguata et al. 2014; Hall et al. 2015; Health and Development Africa 2012; Herman et al. 2009; IDF 2013; Kessler and Bromet 2013; Kessler et al. 2009; Lawn et al. 2006; Lohrmann et al. 2012; Madise et al. 2012; Magadi 2013; Mayosi et al. 2012; Mendenhall et al. 2014; Meyer, Yoon, and Kaufmann 2013; Ministry of Health and Family Welfare 2006; Misra et al. 2001; Mohan et al. 2007; NASCOP 2014; Ndetei et al. 2009; Ogaro et al. 2012; Oti et al. 2013; Oxlade and Murray 2012; Peer et al. 2012; Poongothai et al. 2009; Pratt and Brody 2014; Stein et al. 2008; Ministry of Health & Family Welfare Urban Health Division 2006; WHO 2014.

39. See Leone et al. 2012; Mendenhall et al. 2014.

40. Renn, Feliciano, and Segal 2011 is one example of the growing body of research that argues for the bidirectionality of depression and diabetes, including multiple systematic reviews.

41. See Snoek, Bremmer, and Hermanns (2015, 452); this is part of the *Lancet* Series on Depression and Diabetes comorbidity.

42. See Gomez-Oliver et al. 2014; Nyirenda et al. 2012, 2013; Scholten et al. 2011.

43. See Mugisha et al. 2016. There is increasing movement to add metformin and other diabetes medications to the list of essential medicines that would be provided in global health programming. Although ART has long been on this list (and it has provided impetus to make such a list in the first place), only recently have political movements—mostly among diabetics and the Young Professionals Chronic Disease Network made an impact on increasing access for these essential drugs.

44. There is extensive research now on the relationships of food insecurity (Anema et al. 2014; Himmelgreen et al. 2009) and depression (Sherr et al. 2011)—linked through both social pathways and psychopathology (Guerra et al. 2013)—with HIV/AIDS.

45. For Indonesia, see Alisjahbana et al. 2006; for India, see Kant 2003; for Hispanics in the United States, see Pablos-Méndez, Blustein, and Knirsch 1997; Ponce-De-Leon et al. 2004.

46. See the International Union against Tuberculosis and Lung Disease 2012; Knut, Roglic, and Harries 2014; Lancet Diabetes & Endocrinology 2014.

47. See Riza et al. 2014.

48. See Bateson and Goldsby 1988, 941–44.

49. See Friedman et al. 2015; Herrick et al. 2013; Stall, Friedman, and Catania 2008. Most of the scholarship by Ronald Stall and colleagues is a quantitative analysis and interpretation of syndemic production (as opposed to an experiential, interpretive analysis that is apropos for syndemic suffering). Their work situates risk for HIV into a complex dynamic in which social stigma, social exclusion, and co-occurring conditions among men who have sex with men create what they call "syndemic production." This work suggests that the social world may drive the clustering and interaction of HIV among men who have sex with men as much as any biological interaction that might make the infection more virulent.

50. See Bateson and Goldsby 1988; Farmer 2001; Lindenbaum 1979; Nordstrom 2009; Rhodes et al. 2005.

51. Bateson and Goldsby 1988, cited in Farmer 2001, 182.

52. This concept was first posed by Chambers (1983) but it has been referenced by Merrill Singer, Paul Farmer, and others in relation to AIDS.

53. This is a common term used to talk about high-needs areas in which vulnerable populations facing structural inequalities and health problems are concentrated (see Gawande 2011).

54. I interpret risk through the earlier work of Byron Good (1994), who contends that biomedical approaches to illness do not expose truth, because human experience is affected by multiple levels of social and cultural influence.

55. See Walker, Keane, and Burke 2010.

56. See Basu et al. 2012; Monteiro et al. 2013; Popkin, Adair, and Ng 2012.

2. Chicago

1. Multiple sclerosis is an intense, chronic, and disabling disease that attacks the central nervous system.

2. To qualify for Medicaid, individuals in 2010 must have been making less than $22,050 annually for a family of four, and most women in my study made well below $10,000. Beatriz's income level, which was above this threshold, made her eligible for Medicaid under the Affordable Care Act, although she was not eligible for Medicaid in 2010 when the study was conducted.

3. Marcia Farr's (2006) book, *Rancheros in Chicagoacán*, exemplifies the deeply entangled relationship of Chicagoans with sending communities in Mexico. Farr traces the fluid exchanges of culture and language among a transnational community of *rancheros*—the non-indigenous, non-affluent Mexicans who make up the majority of Mexican immigrants in the United States.

4. See Farr 2006; De Genova and Peutz 2010; Mendenhall 2012; Montoya 2007, 2011.

5. This study was part of a three-phase study of culture, immigration, and health care. In 2006–2007 my colleagues and I conducted an exploratory ethnographic study of Mexican immigrant beliefs about diabetes and experiences living with it. We found that people used their diabetes diagnosis to discuss social distress and disorder in their personal lives, often linking diabetes causality and experience with traumatic and stressful experiences (Mendenhall et al. 2010). These data informed the survey study we conducted in Chicago and San Francisco, specifically examining what cultural and personal factors people linked with diabetes causality; we found that reporting beliefs about traumatic experiences as opposed to strong emotions (e.g., susto [fright] and *coraje* [rage or anger]) was associated with depression (Mendenhall et al. 2012). An in-depth analysis of those women's experiences is published in my first book, *Syndemic Suffering* (Mendenhall 2012).

6. Focusing on low-income people of Mexican descent was a response not only to the growing number of studies at the time that pointed to important links between diabetes and social suffering (Scheder 1988; Schoenberg et al. 2005; Rock 2003, 2005) but also to epidemiological and clinical studies that have long revealed that lifetime risk for diabetes for Mexican Americans is higher (51 percent) than for the general population (40 percent) (Gregg et al. 2014), especially among those who are low-income (see Mezuk et al. 2013). This includes people with diagnosed and undiagnosed diabetes, as it is estimated that only half of those with diabetes have been diagnosed in a clinic. Even more, research on the Latino health paradox reveals the systemic and social factors that undermine immigrants' health, leaving immigrants with more sickness—including depression and diabetes—the longer they reside in the United States (Castaneda et al. 2014).

7. Like in most public clinics, patients at the GMC wait for hours (at least two and sometimes up to six) in a crowded room populated with people from diverse regions of the metropolitan area. A wide variety of languages can be overheard at the GMC, from Spanish to Hindi to some African languages. Official interpreters for twelve languages are spread thin across the hospital, and the GMC alone serves more than 40,000 primary-care visits per year. This is one of one hundred outpatient clinics associated with the 450-bed hospital. Serving the social and psychological needs of all of these patients at the time of this study were eight psychiatrists, two nurse practitioners, four nurses, and three psychologists. The GMC and community-based clinics also often have a social worker on staff to meet the needs of their patients, and some employ an additional nurse counselor or psychologist. When this study

was carried out, one bilingual Spanish-speaking social worker worked within the GMC, and there were two physicians, one nurse, and three psychologists who spoke Spanish in the adjacent psychiatry department. Some clinicians and clerks at the GMC also spoke Spanish, but Spanish-speaking patients were not always paired with them. The unmet needs for Spanish-speaking diabetes care are evident in the fact that 25–30 percent of the patients at the GMC are Latino and 30–40 percent are diabetic. Data on the nationalities of all Latino patients at the GMC are not available, but based on my experience recruiting for various research projects, I estimate that the percentage of people of Mexican descent among all Latinos seeking care at the GMC resembles those of the city at large (75 percent).

8. See Kaiser et al. 2016.

9. Type 2 diabetes is the seventh leading cause of death in the United States, and an estimated 9 percent of the population is affected by it. There is a magnified impact among socially and economically marginalized populations, including American Indians (15.9 percent), Puerto Ricans (14.8 percent), Mexican Americans (13.9 percent), and African Americans (13.2 percent). The latter three groups represent the most affected in Chicago, and there is substantial evidence supporting the link between diabetes and socioeconomic disadvantage in the city (e.g., Ludwig et al. 2011). Similarly, compared to the estimate that around 5 percent of the US population suffer from depression, one in seven people who are poor (14.3 percent) report depressive symptoms (Pratt and Brody 2014).

10. Study participants were compensated $40 for their time; the shortest interview was two hours, the longest interview was six hours, and the average time was around three hours.

11. Life history narrative interviews began with the question: "Can you tell me about your childhood?" Targeted probing included: "Where did you grow up?" and "Can you tell me about your family?" Oftentimes these simple questions launched women into in-depth life stories. If family relationships, emotions, past trauma, mental health, and diabetes management did not come up through the iterative process of qualitative interviewing, we followed up with these key questions: "Have you ever been married?" "What age were your first married? Can you tell me about that relationship?" "Can you tell me about your family, your children?" "Have you ever experienced strong emotions (like rage-anger/coraje)? If so, what caused these emotions?" "Do any emotions affect your diabetes?" "What caused your diabetes?" "How do you manage your diabetes?" and "Have you been depressed or hopeless in the last month?" If a traumatic experience was not mentioned in the interview, then the following question was asked at the end: "Have you experienced any major stress or trauma in your life?" Because our preliminary ethnographic data indicated that gender-based violence was a major issue among socially disadvantaged Mexican-American women, we asked a specific follow-up question if mistreatment or abuse was not mentioned. However, there rarely was a need for follow-up questions, as most women who experienced trauma or mistreatment brought it up during the natural course of the interview.

12. Hemoglobin (Hb) A1c was derived from dried blood spots and analyzed by Flexsite Diagnostics. HbA1c, also known as glycosylated hemoglobin, has become a standard measurement for glycemic control in both clinic- and population-based studies. As Gomero and colleagues (2008) explain, the rationale for this particular biological marker of glycemic control is based on its fairly stable measure over the entire 90–120 day lifespan of the red blood cell. Further, "glycosylated hemoglobin is formed through non-enzymatic binding of circulating glucose to hemoglobin (glycation)" and it "is measured as the ratio of glycosylated to non-glycosylated hemoglobin." As opposed to simply measuring glucose levels at the time of the blood spot or serum measurement, HbA1c may be interpreted as an average of the blood glucose present over the past three to four months.

13. The Center for Epidemiological Studies Depression Scale (CES-D) is a widely used twenty-item questionnaire designed to assess the major symptoms of depression in English

(Radloff 1977), and it has been validated in Spanish (Soler et al. 1997). A reliable and well-validated instrument, the CES-D's targeted symptoms include depressed mood, changes in appetite and sleep, low energy, hopelessness, low self-esteem, and loneliness. Respondents were asked to consider the presence and duration of each item/symptom over the past week and to rate each along a four-point scale from 0 (rarely or never) to 3 (most or all of the time). Possible CES-D scores range from 0 to 60. Scores ≥16 have been validated for use as a screen for "likely depression" in the community population, and scores ≥24 have been recommended to screen for depression in the clinical population.

14. I measured post-traumatic stress disorder by administering the PTSD-Checklist Civilian Version (PCL-C). The PCL-C is a widely used seventeen-item questionnaire designed to assess key symptoms of PTSD in the general population in both English and Spanish (Miles, Marshall, and Schell 2008). A reliable and freely available instrument adapted from the PCL-M (checklist used for the military), it lists as key symptoms of PTSD: repeated, disturbing memories and dreams; feeling as though the stressful event were happening again; feeling upset and having physical reactions to events that elicit memories of the past; trouble sleeping and remembering events; feeling distant from family and friends; and feeling jumpy or hypervigilant. These seventeen symptoms were taken directly from the DSM criteria. Respondents were asked to consider presence and duration of each symptom over the past month and to rate each along a five-point scale from 1 (not at all) to 5 (extremely). Possible scores ranged from 17 to 85. A score ≥30 is the recommended cutoff point indicating a PTSD diagnosis in a civilian primary care setting, as opposed to the screening cutoff point of 25 for combat veterans. Scores <30 were considered "no or few symptoms."

15. Anthropometrics, including height and weight, were collected at the end of the interview, and body mass index was generated based on these measurements. Waist circumference was also measured using a standard seamstress tape measure. Systolic and diastolic blood pressures were evaluated employing a standard blood pressure monitor used in the medical setting.

16. I also evaluated links of stressors to cultural idioms, but they were not significant. I believe this was due to the fact that I did not use a locally derived distress scale. Others, such as Susan Weller and colleagues (2008), have found that *nervios* and susto are associated with depression.

17. Stress related to finances, family, work, immigration, and neighborhood violence were not significantly associated with depression in these analyses. Next, I took this one step further to investigate if these narrative forms of distress that increased the odds of depression interacted among themselves. I conducted multivariate analyses to better understand what was at play in the potentially powerful link between interpersonal abuse and depression. There was significant evidence in this analysis showing that interpersonal abuse significantly predicted depression after adjusting for health stress and diabetes stress, both alone and taken together. This finding reflects the entanglements of such violence with the pervasiveness of financial, social, and personal stresses through the life course.

18. This figure was first published in Mendenhall 2012, 106.

19. Psychiatric inventories indicated that she had symptoms of PTSD (PCL-C: 32) and severe depression (CES-D: 30).

20. A study among low-income and undocumented women in California reports similar findings (Heilemann, Kury, and Lee 2005); another study demonstrates that intra-ethnic differentiation matters because it underscores the precarity and risk that low-income women face (Lown and Vega 2001).

21. See Finkler 1994, 1997; Gutmann 1999; Hirsch 2003; Holmes 2013.

22. See Baker et al. 2009; Heilemann, Kury, and Lee 2005; Lown and Vega 2001.

23. See Hunt, Schneider, and Comer 2004.

24. See Castaneda 2010; Castaneda et al. 2014.
25. See Farr 2006; Finkler 1994; Hirsch 2003.
26. See Fisher et al. 2000.

3. Delhi

1. Many people residing in Delhi today relocated after the Partition of British India in 1947 into India and Pakistan, which in many cases created a major migration of Muslims to Pakistan and of Hindus to India. Delhi has been continuously inhabited since the sixth century, serving as the capital of myriad kingdoms and empires. With the rise and fall of each, Delhi has been destroyed and rebuilt, resulting in a combination of small cities spread out and unified through a metropolitan region. New Delhi, which is the capital seat of India, is a smaller geographic region within the Delhi metropolitan area, and it represents only one of eleven districts, with just over 250,000 residents.

2. The National Heart, Lung, and Blood Institute (NHLBI) at the National Institutes of Health in Bethesda, Maryland, has supported the development of multiple Centers of Excellence in low- and middle-income countries (LMIC). Such centers support partnerships between US and LMIC researchers and foster research that builds capacity for improved understanding of noncommunicable diseases. The Delhi COE-CARRS partnership is with Emory University, and it is led by Dr. K. M. Venkat Narayan at the Global Diabetes Center. See http://www.nhlbi.nih.gov/about/org/globalhealth/centers/new-delhi-center-of-excellence.htm.

3. The in-depth interview was modified from the one used for the Chicago study. The questions about early childhood were moved to a second section and the interview began with questions about daily life. Many of the modifications were intended to make our interlocutors feel more at ease and were made in discussion with my mentors at PHFI and Emory University as well as the local research staff and my research assistants. The interview was piloted with the research staff and modified significantly over the period of one month. Once completed and situated within the Indian cultural context, in accordance with the priorities of the CARRS research team, the qualitative interview was completed in English, translated into Hindi, and back-translated into English. Each narrative interview began with: "Can you describe a typical day for me?" The interview then shifted to address the study participants' understanding of and experiences with stress, including questions like, "What does stress mean to you?" and "Have you experienced a stressful situation in the past 30 days? Can you describe it? What aspects of your life cause you the most tension?" Because the English term "tension" is commonly used to express stressful experiences in India (Weaver and Hadley 2011), we often probed using the terms "tension" and "stress" interchangeably. We also asked targeted questions about social relationships, including family and community tensions or support systems. We spent the last half of the interview discussing issues associated with diabetes, including questions like, "What caused your diabetes?" "Has diabetes changed your life in any way?" "Has diabetes affected your daily routine?" and "Does stress or tension affect your diabetes in any way?" Finally, we asked a number of questions about diabetes management, such as, "Can you tell me about how you care for your diabetes?" "Who makes decisions about your diabetes care?" and "Where do you seek diabetes care? And how often?"

4. The Hopkins Symptoms Checklist (HSCL-25) is a twenty-five-item questionnaire in which respondents are asked to score each mood-related item on a scale ranging from 0 ("not at all") to 3 ("extremely"). The HSCL-25 was selected because it was validated in Hindi by another team of anthropologists (Weaver and Hadley 2011). The depression component of the HSCL (questions 11–25) was averaged over the number of items, and a score greater than 1.75 was considered a clinically significant level of depression.

5. See Mendenhall et al. 2012b, p. 2526. Please refer to table 3, where these differences are described in detail.

6. Common biomedical tropes foster a dominant discourse of patient autonomy and responsibility, pointing to individual responsibility and self-control as proximate causes and cures for diseases (Browne et al. 2013; Schabert et al. 2013; Seligman et al. 2015). Browne and colleagues (2013) have argued that biomedical practice commonly places blame on the ill for developing diabetes and for failing to prevent diabetes complications. As a result, people with diabetes often feel stigma imbued with moral blame, shame, and guilt (see Broom and Whittaker 2004). This was documented in Australia, where researchers found that 84 percent of people with diabetes reported social stigma and personal (or self-perpetuated) stigma (Browne et al. 2013). In research with Mexican Americans with diabetes, we found that people develop burdensome feelings of stress and moral blame associated with the failure to adhere to the physicians' expectations for self-care (Seligman et al. 2015).

7. See Fernandes 2004.

8. See Marrow 2013.

9. Refer to seminal writing in anthropology on the household as the locus of culture and morals, such as Lévi-Strauss 1969.

10. See Das Gupta 1995.

11. Vikram Patel and colleagues at Sangath (a nonprofit health institution in Goa, India) have written extensively on the intersectional complexities of gender, income, and mental health care (Andrew et al. 2012; Patel et al. 1998; Patel, Rodrigues, and DeSouza 2002). Another good paper on gender, household, and mental health reveals how women's social and familial experiences cannot be dissociated rom mental health (Chokkanathan 2009).

12. The social obligation of dowry (Anderson 2003) and the crippling effects of dowry on low-income families (see Mankekar 1998) have transformed substantially in recent decades.

13. The anthropologists Veena Das (1997) and Lesley Jo Weaver (2016) have described in detail how the interpersonal suffering of women within the family plays an important role in society.

14. See Snell-Rood 2015.

15. See Weaver et al. 2015.

16. Medical anthropologists have been accused of occupying the suffering slot (Butt 2002; Herrick 2017), a critique that suggests that focusing too much on suffering obfuscates possibilities for determining sources of resilience that are cultural, social, or political. In many ways, the syndemics literature to date is guilty of occupying this domain—and there is a great deal of opportunity to flip it around. Sara Lewis's (2013, 2018) scholarship among Tibetan refugees in northern India, for example, suggests that the cultural practice of compassion, meditation, and letting go of negative emotions may reduce psychological symptomatology, even in the face of extraordinary suffering. She argues that, as opposed to framing things in terms of trauma, Tibetan Buddhists employ a shared cultural understanding framed by Buddhist doctrine whereby people do not reject but instead reframe loss, violence, and displacement. She does not argue that this is a potential source for mental health intervention (which is an attractive interpretation, especially given the increasing interest of the medical field for innovative ways to promote mental health across diverse contexts); instead, she suggests that this cultural practice reveals a form of agency through which people recapture power denied to them.

4. Soweto

1. The cultural idiom of "thinking too much" is both inclusive of local idioms of distress and overlapping with global idioms of stress and depression. Some of the earliest work on thinking too much in Zimbabwe, known as *kufungisisa* in the Shona language, revealed that the idiom communicated how people related distress to a supernatural cause or social stressor (Patel et al. 1995a, 1995b). This work spurred debate in part because Patel and colleagues

(2001) argued that thinking too much demonstrated a significant overlap with depression and anxiety that might warrant utilizing the construct in biomedical diagnoses. Their argument was met with criticism by those who argued that the psychiatric utilization of cultural concepts often reifies culture, constructing it as a static reality rather than a fluid and interactive construct shaped by history, politics, and society (Jenkins 2015; Kirmayer 2012). Today, "thinking too much" is one of the most commonly catalogued idioms of distress, represented globally in ethnographic studies and included as one of the cultural idioms in the DSM-5 (Kaiser et al. 2015; Kohrt et al. 2014).

2. For a more lucid exploration of these concepts, see Comaroff and Comaroff 1991, 1999.

3. See Lewis 1966.

4. My thinking about what these political categories of "race" mean was shaped by my dialogue with Linda Richter at the South African Human Sciences Research Council and by the work of Ellison and colleagues (1997). I use the political category of "Black" to describe the women in this study because it has social significance within South Africa, despite the problematic history of the term. Categories of "Black," "White," and "Coloured" were used during apartheid to differentiate groups from one another and have become common ways in which people self-identify. However, these terms do not reflect the ethnic diversity within South Africa, as those who self-identify as Black may speak different languages within the home, identify with different ethnic groups, and relay to family in different regions.

5. "The history of Soweto has been marked by a progressive collapse of a state authority, an often violent struggle against representatives of the state . . . a breakdown of paternal authority within families . . . and the general rise in crime and insecurity" (Ashforth 1995, cited in Hansen 2011).

6. See Richter et al. 2007. Birth to Twenty Plus is one of multiple cohort studies meant to study the developmental origins hypothesis that have expanded exponentially to capture changing physical landscapes through time.

7. For a good analysis of how these political-economic changes affected health, refer to the South Africa Series published in the *Lancet* in 2009 (Chopra et al. 2009; Coovadia et al. 2009; Karim et al. 2009; Mayosi et al. 2009; Peltzer 2009; Seedat et al. 2009).

8. The narrative interview was inspired by the studies in Chicago and Delhi but extensively revised based on discussions with the research staff and key researchers involved in the Birth to Twenty study as well as piloting with research staff who resided in Soweto or similar low-income neighborhoods in Johannesburg. Each narrative interview began with "Can you describe a typical day?" The interview then shifted to address women's understanding of and experiences with stress, including questions like "What does stress mean to you?" "How do you define stress?" and "What aspects of your life cause you the most stress?" We also asked targeted questions about family and community relationships and support systems. We spent the last half of the interview discussing diabetes, including questions like "Has diabetes changed your life in any way?" and "Does stress affect your diabetes in any way?" We also inquired about their perceptions of the relationships among multiple morbidities. We concluded the interview with questions around health care experiences and a short survey of previously diagnosed disorders, including obesity, hypertension, anxiety, depression, HIV, tuberculosis, and arthritis.

9. The CES-D was selected because it had been previously utilized in my study in Chicago as well as by DPHRU.

10. All interviews were audio-recorded, and women were compensated 50 ZAR (around $5.88) for transportation costs. All data collection received clearance by the University of the Witwatersrand Human Ethics Committee.

11. HIV prevalence in South Africa was reported by the South African HIV Prevalence and Behavioral Survey of 2012 to be 12 percent, with higher rates among women (14.4 percent)

compared to men (9.9 percent); Black Africans (15 percent) compared to Whites (0.3 percent), Coloureds (3.1 percent), and Indians/Asians (0.8 percent); and those residing in urban informal settlements (19.9 percent) compared to urban formal (10.1 percent), rural formal (10.4 percent), and rural informal (13.4 percent) settlements. The most affected group were people between thirty and forty years of age, with a prevalence around 40 percent. HIV prevalence drops sharply as the population ages, with only 3 percent of people affected who are older than 60 years of age; most likely this is because people do not live to this age with the virus. See Shisana et al. 2012.

12. See Fassin 2007, 24.

13. See Tregenna and Tsela 2012.

14. See Hoogeveen and Özler 2005.

15. See Walker, Keane, and Burke 2010. This review highlights how food deserts have been a subject of extensive research in the United States and exemplifies the concept of structural violence, whereby systematic inequalities impede people's abilities to maintain healthy diets due to lack of accessibility and affordability.

16. See Battersby 2011, 2012. The food insecurity of urban South Africans is significant because, as Battersby argues, development priorities and national priorities about food security emphasize the needs of the rural poor, often overlooking the severity of food insecurity in urban areas.

17. See Cannuscio, Weiss, and Asch 2010.

18. See Ruel-Bergeron et al. 2015, as well as Moran-Thomas 2012.

19. See Posel and Rogan 2012. This trend was most prominent when contrasting households led by women with households led by to men.

20. See Seedat et al. 2009.

21. See Peden, McGee, and Sharma 2002.

22. See Dunkle et al. 2004.

23. This is not surprising, given the legacy of violence linked to tsotsis (gangs) in Soweto (see Glaser 2008).

24. Seedat et al. 2009 provides details about who perpetrates homicide and who is victimized by it.

25. See Mendenhall et al. 2013. In this study we used the General Health Questionnaire (GHQ) -28 to evaluate psychological morbidity, which included somatic symptoms, anxiety, depression, and social dysfunction. The 45 percent reporting of psychological morbidity across the sample (n = 1,743) reflects more somatic and anxiety symptoms than depressive symptoms.

26. See Gradidge et al. 2016. This was analyzed among the Birth to Twenty caregivers.

27. See Wood and Lambert 2008.

28. See Le Marcis 2012.

29. See Black 2012.

30. See Zuch and Lurie 2012.

31. These ideas were formulated in conversation with the medical anthropologist Lesley Jo Weaver on the occasion of our presentation on "Catch-All Stigma in India and South Africa" at the American Anthropological Association meeting in Minneapolis, MN, November 16–20, 2016.

5. Nairobi

1. See Mendenhall et al. 2019.

2. See Ekdale 2004.

3. See Muwonge 1980.

4. See Huchzermeyer 2008.

5. See Davis 2006.

6. See APHRC 2014.

7. We used the Beck Depression Inventory (BDI-II) (Beck, Steer, and Brown 1996) and the Beck Anxiety Inventory (BAI) (Beck and Steer 1990) in this study because it was commonly used and had been translated by the AMHF. The BDI-II and BAI are common tools used to index depression and anxiety symptomatology. These psychiatric inventories were validated in Kenya for people seeking primary care by my colleagues David Ndetei and Victoria Mutiso from the Africa Mental Health Foundation, and demonstrated corresponding cutoffs (Ndetei et al. 2010). For depression, twenty-one BDI-II items were evaluated along a four-point scale (from 0 to 3, from symptoms never reported to symptoms present most of the time). These scores were summed to provide a single score for minimal (0–13), mild (14–19), moderate (20–28), and severe (29–63) depression. For anxiety, twenty-one BAI items were evaluated with a four-point scale (from 0 to 3, from symptoms not bothering the respondents at all to symptoms bothering them a lot). The sum of these scores provides a single score for minimal (1–21), moderate (22–35), and severe (36–63) anxiety.

8. See Bor et al. 2013.

9. Refer to the work of the African Population and Health Research Center, focused on health and livelihoods in slums (APHRC 2014).

10. See de Smedt 2011.

11. See Mendenhall et al. 2015, 15, Table 2.

12. See Joireman and Vanderpoel 2008.

13. See APHRC 2014.

14. See Cooper 2011.

15. See Kimuna and Kjamba 2008.

16. See Swart 2011.

17. See Mutahi 2011.

18. See Hajjebrahimi et al. 2016; also refer to the multiple chapters on the psychophysiology of fear in Kirmayer, Lemelson, and Barad 2007.

19. See Gallaher et al. 2013.

20. See Mendenhall et al. 2015.

21. See Needham and Hill 2010.

22. See Preiss, Brennan, and Clarke 2013.

23. See Holt, Groot, and Golden 2014.

24. See Mendenhall et al. 2013. This article was written with colleagues from the Birth to Twenty Plus study to illustrate how impactful increasing physical morbidities are on the mental health of caregivers in the Birth to Twenty Plus cohort.

25. See Hulzebosch et al. 2015.

26. See Yuen et al. 2014.

27. See Atun and Gale 2015; Baker et al. 2011; Riza et al. 2014.

28. See Butt et al. 2009.

29. See Goudge et al. 2009; Mendenhall and Norris 2015a.

30. See, for example, Gilson and McIntyre 2005.

31. See Opwora et al. 2015.

32. See Hercot et al. 2011; Kien et al. 2016.

Conclusion

1. See Benton 2015; Kenworthy 2017; Kenworthy and Parker 2014; Kenworthy and Thomann 2017; Shiffman 2008. Over the first three decades of the HIV/AIDS epidemic, funding continued to escalate with great fervor, with the majority of it earmarked for those infected with HIV, transforming the crisis into a somewhat controlled epidemic (employing

treatment as prevention). Although HIV/AIDS programming was explicitly vertical, it also exemplified what many call a diagonal program through which HIV/AIDS funding may elevate the health system (by way of building laboratories and training staff, as examples). Nevertheless, in many cases, those with HIV experienced distinct privileges and access to resources within the health system. Yet, since the 2008 recession, we have observed a scaling down of AIDS programming as a direct result of reduction in funding. This affected not only HIV/AIDS funding but also global health as a form of development more broadly.

2. See Bommer et al. 2017; Daniels, Donilon, and Bollyky 2014. The latter reference is a special report published by the Council on Foreign Relations that underscored the looming economic impact of the non-communicable disease epidemics in poor countries, due in part to the sluggish response by the international community. Refer also to the recent articles by the *Lancet* Taskforce on NCDs and Economics on the economics of ignoring diabetes in low- and middle-income countries (Jan et al. 2018; Niessen et al. 2018; Nugent et al. 2018; Sassi et al. 2018).

3. See IDF 2015. According to this source, 12 percent of the current global health expenditure is dedicated to diabetes treatment and related complications, and the majority of this expenditure is located in the United States ($320 billion), followed by China, which spends significantly less ($51 billion). Comparatively, the United States has 29.3 million people with diabetes (ranking third globally), compared to China, which has the greatest affliction ($109.6 million), and India, which is second ($69.2 million). The list of the ten most afflicted countries (China, India, United States, Brazil, Russian Federation, Mexico, Indonesia, Egypt, Japan, and Bangladesh) does not coincide with the list of the top ten countries or territories by health-care expenditure (United States, China, Germany, Japan, Brazil, France, Russian Federation, United Kingdom, and Italy).

4. See Popkin 2006; Popkin 2015; Popkin, Adair, Ng, 2012; Popkin & Hawkes 2015.

5. See Yates-Doerr 2015.

6. See Marshall 2014.

7. See also Taubes 2016.

8. See Nestle 2013; Patel 2012. Big Food refers to those corporations that profit immensely through exploitive practice, preying on and taking advantage of vulnerable consumers and producers in the global food and agricultural system.

9. In *The Unending Hunger*, Megan Carney (2015) poignantly describes the biopolitics of food insecurity, showing how hidden sugars in Big Food products compound the gendered complexities of immigration and stress that cultivate diabetes and obesity syndemically among Mexican immigrants like María.

10. See Battersby 2012, 146.

11. See Thayer and Non 2015.

12. See Kuzawa and Quinn 2009.

13. This argument relies on the extensive literature on global mental health and the growing literature on diabetes and psychosocial health. On global mental health, see Chatterjee et al. 2008; Kakuma et al. 2011; Lund et al. 2010, 2012; Lund, Tomlinson, and Patel 2015; Patel et al. 2011. On diabetes and psychosocial health, see Beaglehole et al. 2008; Daniel et al. 1999; García-Huidobro et al. 2011; Joshi et al. 2014; Talbot and Nouwen 2000; Walker et al. 2015; Werfalli et al. 2015.

14. See Thayer et al. 2016.

15. See Seligman et al. 2015; also refer to note 6 from chapter 3.

16. See Parsons 1951.

17. See Weaver 2016.

18. For a more extensive discussion, see Manderson and Smith-Morris 2010; Seeberg and Meinert 2015.

19. See the *Lancet* Taskforce on NCDs and Economics led by Rachel Nugent, which has produced the most recent collection of papers linking household and national economics with NCDs and stressing the need to address foods, drinks, and tobacco as sources of poor health (Jan et al. 2018; Niessen et al. 2018; Nugent et al. 2018; Sassi et al. 2018).

20. See Arthur Kleinman's extensive work and reference to "what's at stake" when attempting to understand sociopolitical contexts and the moral predicaments of patients and sufferers (Kleinman 1986, 1995, 1999). This was also discussed in Kirmayer 2006.

21. See Jan et al. 2018.

22. See Wilkinson and Pickett 2011, which provides a comprehensive argument of how and why wealth and health inequalities are tightly aligned.

23. It is worth taking a closer look at the body of scholarship produced by David Stuckler and Sanjay Basu, especially their book *The Body Economic: Why Austerity Kills* (Stuckler and Basu 2013). See also Alleyne et al. 2013; Basu et al. 2012, 2014; Vellakkal et al. 2013, 2014; Yach, Stuckler, and Brownell 2006.

24. See Nestle 2013, 2015.

25. See WHO 2007.

26. See Balabanova et al. 2013; Gilson and Millsb 1995; Makinen et al. 2000.

27. See Goudge et al. 2009.

28. See Hercot et al. 2011.

29. See for example Balabanova et al. 2013.

30. See Dye et al. 2013.

31. See Farmer et al. 2013 for a good overview.

32. See Clinton and Sridhar 2017.

33. See Joshi et al. 2014; Petersen et al. 2012; WHO 2008.

34. See Quigley 2009. See also http://www.ampathkenya.org/.

35. See Mamlin et al. 2009.

36. See Monahan et al. 2009.

37. See Pastakia et al. 2013.

38. See Kidder et al. 2011.

39. See Bourgois et al. 2017.

40. See also Weaver and Hadley 2011.

41. See Prince et al. 2007.

42. See Bolton et al. 2003.

43. See Gawande 2011.

44. See Emeche 2015.

45. One good example of a useful app is the Trever Project in DC, which has an app targeting LGBTQ youth to mitigate crises, especially suicide (see https://www.thetrevorproject.org). Another good example is MindRight (see https://getmindright.org/welcome), which is a "judgement-free place for growing, healing, and hope" where youth of color can text or call to receive support. Participants can text coaches before and after school, and coaches check in daily to make sure participants are doing okay. Some weeks may involve only a quick check-in if everything is okay, and other weeks may involve more intensive coaching as youth face various stressors and challenges.

46. Refer to Rahman et al. 2008a, 2008b; Singla, Kumbakumba, and Aboud 2015.

47. See Maes 2016. An important issue to heed, however, is that a syndemic care model should be comprehensively implemented in order to prevent overburdening community health workers with extra tasks. With the increasing distribution of tasks to community health workers, there is a growing concern about lack of compensation and workers' physical and mental health problems (Maes 2015; Maes et al. 2015b). This is especially problematic given that the

majority of community health workers are women and thus bear the greatest burden of uncompensated or undercompensated labor (Closser 2015; Maes et al. 2015a).

48. See http://www.philips.com/a-w/foundation/philips-foundation.html.

49. See also Hardin 2015, 2018.

50. See examples from the fields of HIV care (McGuire et al. 2013) and mental health care (Padmanathan and DeSilva 2013).

51. See WHO 2008.

References

Agardh, Emilie, Peter Allebeck, Johan Hallqvist, Tahereh Moradi, and Anna Sidorchuk. 2011. "Type 2 Diabetes Incidence and Socio-Economic Position: A Systematic Review and Meta-Analysis." *International Journal of Epidemiology* 40: 804–18.

Ahlqvist, Emma, Petter Storm, Annemari Käräjämäki, Mats Martinell, Mozhgan Dorkhan, Annelie Carlsson, Petter Vikman, et al. 2018. "Novel Subgroups of Adult-Onset Diabetes and Their Association with Outcomes: A Data-Driven Cluster Analysis of Six Variables." *Lancet Diabetes & Endocrinology* 6 (5): 361–69.

Alisjahbana, B., R. van Crevel, E. Sahiratmadja, M. den Heijer, and A. Mayua. 2006. "Diabetes Mellitus Is Strongly Associated with Tuberculosis in Indonesia." *International Journal of Tuberculosis and Lung Disease* 10: 696–700.

Alleyne, George, Agnes Binagwaho, Andy Haines, Selim Jahan, Rachel Nugent, Ariella Rojhani, David Stuckler, and Lancet NCD Action Group. 2013. "Embedding Non-Communicable Diseases in the Post-2015 Development Agenda." *Lancet* 381 (9866): 566–74.

American Diabetes Association. 2014. "National Diabetes Statistics Report, 2009–2012, 2014 Estimates of Diabetes and Its Burden in the Epidemiologic Estimation Methods." National Center for Chronic Disease Prevention and Health Promotion, Centers for Disease Control. Atlanta, GA.

Anderson, Siwan. 2003. "Why Dowry Payments Declined with Modernization in Europe but Are Rising in India." *Journal of Political Economy* 111 (2): 269–310.

Andrew, Gracy, Alex Cohen, Shruti Salgaonkar, and Vikram Patel. 2012. "The Explanatory Models of Depression and Anxiety in Primary Care: A Qualitative Study from India." *BMC Research Notes* 12 (5): 499.

Anema, Aranka, Sarah J. Fielden, Tony Castleman, Nils Grede, Amie Heap, and Martin Bloem. 2014. "Food Security in the Context of HIV: Towards Harmonized Definitions and Indicators." *AIDS and Behavior* 18 (Suppl. 5): 476–89.

APHRC (African Population and Health Research Center). 2014. "Population and Health Dynamics in Nairobi's Informal Settlements: Report of the Nairobi Cross-Sectional Slums Survey (NCSS) 2012." Nairobi, Kenya: APHRC.

Appadurai, Arjun. 1986. "Theory in Anthropology: Center and Periphery." *Comparative Studies in Society and History* 28 (2): 356–61.

———. 1996. *Modernity at Large: Cultural Dimensions of Globalization.* Minneapolis: University of Minnesota Press.

Ashforth, Adam. 1995, Mar 2. "State Power, Violence, Everyday Life: Soweto." Working Paper No. 210, Center for the Study of Social Change (CSSC) working papers, 1985–1998. New School Archives and Special Collections, The New School, New York, New York.

Atun, Rifat, and Edwin A. M. Gale. 2015. "The Challenge of Diabetes in Sub-Saharan Africa." *Lancet Diabetes & Endocrinology* 3 (9): 675–77.

Ayah, Richard, Mark D. Joshi, Rosemary Wanjiru, Elijah K. Njau, C. Fredrick Otieno, Erastus K. Njeru, and Kenneth K. Mutai. 2013. "A Population-Based Survey of Prevalence of Diabetes and Correlates in an Urban Slum Community in Nairobi, Kenya." *BMC Public Health* 13: 371.

Baker, Charlene K, Fran H. Norris, Eric C. Jones, and Arthur D. Murphy. 2009. "Childhood Trauma and Adulthood Physical Health in Mexico." *Journal of Behavioral Medicine* 32 (3): 255–69.

Baker, Jack, Magdalena Hurtado, Osbjorn Pearson, and Troy Jones. 2008. "Evolutionary Medicine and Obesity: Developmental Adaptive Responses in Human Body Composition." In *Evolutionary Medicine and Health*, edited by Wenda R. Trevathan, E. O. Smith, and James J. McKenna, 314–24. Oxford, UK: Oxford University Press.

Baker, Meghan A., Anthony D. Harries, Christie Y. Jeon, Jessica E. Hart, Anil Kapur, Knut Lönnroth, Salah-Eddine Ottmani, Sunali D. Goonesekera, and Megan B. Murray. 2011. "The Impact of Diabetes on Tuberculosis Treatment Outcomes: A Systematic Review." *BMC Medicine* 9 (1): 81.

Balabanova, Dina, Anne Mills, Lesong Conteh, Baktygul Akkazieva, Hailom Banteyerga, Umakant Dash, Lucy Gilson, Andrew Harmer, Ainura Ibraimova, Ziaul Islam, et al. 2013. "Good Health at Low Cost 25 Years on: Lessons for the Future." *Lancet* 381 (9883): 2118–33.

Barker, David J. 1995. "Fetal Origins of Coronary Heart Disease." *BMJ* 311: 171–74.

———. 1999. "Fetal Origins of Type 2 Diabetes Mellitus." *Annual Review of Internal Medicine* 130: 322–24.

Barker, David J., Paul D. Winter, Clive Osmond, Barrie Margetts, and Shirley J. Simmonds. 1989. "Weight in Infancy and Death from Ischaemic Heart Disease." *Lancet* 2: 577–80.

Basso, Keith. 1996. *Wisdom Sits in Places: Landscape and Language among the Western Apache.* Albuquerque: University of New Mexico Press.

Basu, Sanjay, David Stuckler, Martin McKee, and Gauden Galea. 2012. "Nutritional Determinants of Worldwide Diabetes: An Econometric Study of Food Markets and Diabetes Prevalence in 173 Countries—Corrigendum." *Public Health Nutrition* 16 (1): 1.

Basu, Sanjay, Sukumar Vellakkal, Sutapa Agrawal, David Stuckler, Barry Popkin, and Shah Ebrahim. 2014. "Averting Obesity and Type 2 Diabetes in India through Sugar-Sweetened Beverage Taxation: An Economic-Epidemiologic Modeling Study." *PLoS Medicine* 11 (1): e1001582.

Bateson, Mary Catherine, and Richard A. Goldsby. 1988. *Thinking AIDS: The Social Response to the Biological Threat*. Reading, MA: Addison-Wesley.

Battersby, Jane. 2011. "Urban Food Insecurity in Cape Town, South Africa: An Alternative Approach to Food Access." *Development Southern Africa* 28 (4): 545–61.

———. 2012. "Beyond the Food Desert: Finding Ways to Speak About Urban Food Security in South Africa." *Geografiska Annaler: Series B, Human Geography* 94 (2): 141–59.

Beaglehole, Robert Epping-Jordan, JoAnne, Vikram Patel, Mickey Chopra, Shah Ebrahim, Michael Kidd, and Andy Haines. 2008. "Improving the Prevention and Management of Chronic Disease in Low-Income and Middle-Income Countries: A Priority for Primary Health Care." *Lancet* 372 (9642): 940–49.

Beagley, Jessica, Leonor Guariguata, Clara Weil, and Ayesha A. Motala. 2013. "Global Estimates of Undiagnosed Diabetes in Adults." *Diabetes Research and Clinical Practice* 103 (2): 150–60.

Beck, Aaron T., Steer Robert A. 1990. *Manual for the Beck Anxiety Inventory*. San Antonio, TX: Psychological Corporation.

Beck, Aaron T., Steer Robert A., Brown Gregory K. 1996. *Manual for the BDI-II*. San Antonio, TX: Psychological Corporation.

Becker, Gay. 1997. *Disrupted Lives: How People Create Meaning in a Chaotic World*. Berkeley: University of California Press.

Behar, Ruth. 2003. *Translated Woman: Crossing the Border with Esperanza's Story*. New York: Beacon.

Benton, Adia. 2015. *HIV Exceptionalism: Development through Disease in Sierra Leone*. Minneapolis: University of Minnesota Press.

Berkman, Lisa F., and Ichiro Kawachi, eds. 2000. *Social Epidemiology*. New York: Oxford University Press.

Berkman, Lisa F., and S. Leonard Syme. 1979. "Social Networks, Host Resistance and Mortality: A Nine-Year Follow-up of Alameda County Residents." *American Journal of Epidemiology* 109: 186–204.

Berkman, Lisa F., Thomas Glass, Ian Brissette, and Teresa E Seeman. 2000. "From Social Integration to Health: Durkheim in the New Millennium." *Social Science & Medicine* 51 (6): 843–57.

Bernard, Russell. 2006. *Research Methods in Anthropology: Qualitative and Quantitative Approaches*. Lanham, MD: AltaMira. 4th ed.

Biehl, João. 2005. *VITA: Life in a Zone of Social Abandonment*. Berkeley: University of California Press.

———. 2007. *Will to Live: AIDS Therapies and the Politics of Survival*. Princeton, NJ: Princeton University Press.

Black, Steven P. 2012. "Laughing to Death: Joking as Support amid Stigma for Zulu-Speaking South Africans Living with HIV." *Journal of Linguistic Anthropology* 22 (1): 87–108.

Boehm, Deborah A. 2012. *Intimate Migrations: Gender, Family, and Illegality among Transnational Mexicans.* New York: New York University Press.

Bolton, Paul, Judith Bass, Helen Verdeli, Kathleen F Clougherty, and Lincoln Ndogoni. 2003. "Group Interpersonal Psychotherapy for Depression in Rural Uganda: Randomized Controlled Trial." *JAMA* 289 (23): 3117–24.

Bommer, Christian, Esther Heesemann, Vera Sagalova, Jennifer Manne-Goehler, Rifat Atun, Till Bärnighausen, and Sebastian Vollmer. 2017. "The Global Economic Burden of Diabetes in Adults Aged 20–79 Years: A Cost-of-Illness Study." *Lancet Diabetes & Endocrinology* 5 (6): 423–30.

Bor, Jacob, Abraham J. Herbst, Marie-Louise Newell, and Till Bärnighausen. 2013. "Increases in Adult Life Expectancy in Rural South Africa: Valuing the Scale-Up of HIV Treatment." *Science* 339 (6122): 961–65.

Bourdieu, Pierre, and Loïc Wacquant. 2004. "Symbolic Violence." In *War and Peace: An Anthology*, edited by Nancy Scheper-Hughes and Philippe Bourgois, 272–74. Malden, MA: Blackwell Publishing.

Bourgois, Philippe. 2001. "The Power of Violence in War and Peace: Post-Cold War Lessons from El Salvador." *Ethnography* 2 (1): 5–34.

——. 2009. "Recognizing Invisible Violence." In *Global Health in Times of Violence*, edited by Barbara Rylko-Bauer, Linda Whiteford, and Paul Farmer, 17–40. Santa Fe, NM: School for Advanced Research Press.

Bourgois, Philippe, Seth M. Holmes, Kim Sue, and James Quesada. 2017. "Structural Vulnerability: Operationalizing the Concept to Address Health Disparities in Clinical Care." *Academic Medicine* 92 (3): 299–307.

Broom, Dorothy, and Andrea Whittaker. 2004. "Controlling Diabetes, Controlling Diabetics: Moral Language in the Management of Diabetes Type 2." *Social Science & Medicine* 58: 2371–82.

Browne, Jessica L., Adriana Ventura, Kylie Mosely, and Jane Speight. 2013. "'I Call It the Blame and Shame Disease': A Qualitative Study about Perceptions of Social Stigma Surrounding Type 2 Diabetes." *BMJ Open* 3 (11): e003384.

Butt, Adeel A., Kathleen McGinnis, Maria C. Rodriguez-Barradas, Stephen Crystal, Michael Simberkoff, Matthew Bidwell Goetz, David Leaf, Amy C Justice, and Veterans Aging Cohort Study. 2009. "HIV Infection and the Risk of Diabetes Mellitus." *AIDS* 23 (10): 1227–34.

Butt, Leslie. 2002. "The Suffering Stranger: Medical Anthropology and International Morality." *Medical Anthropology: Cross-Cultural Studies in Health and Illness* 21 (1): 1–24.

Bygbjerg, Ib Christian 2012. "Double Burden of Noncommunicable and Infectious Diseases in Developing Countries." *Science* 337: 1499–501.

Cannuscio, Carolyn C., Eve E. Weiss, and David A. Asch. 2010. "The Contribution of Urban Foodways to Health Disparities." *Journal of Urban Health* 87 (3): 381–93.

Carney, Megan. 2015. *The Unending Hunger: Tracing Women and Food Insecurity across Borders.* Berkeley: University of California Press.

Carruth, Lauren, and Emily Mendenhall. 2018. "Social Aetiologies of Type 2 Diabetes." *BMJ* 361: k1795.

Casqueiro, Juliana, Janine Casqueiro, and Cresio Alves. 2012. "Infections in Patients with Diabetes Mellitus: A Review of Pathogenesis." *Indian Journal of Endocrinology and Metabolism* 16 (Suppl. 1): S27.

Castaneda, Heide. 2010. "Im/Migration and Health: Conceptual, Methodological, and Theoretical Propositions for Applied Anthropology." *NAPA Bulletin* 34: 6–27.

Castaneda, Heide, Seth M. Holmes, Daniel S. Madrigal, Maria-elena Detrinidad Young, Naomi Beyeler, and James Quesada. 2014. "Immigration as a Social Determinant of Health." *Annual Review of Public Health* 36: 1–18.

CBHSQ (Center for Behavioral Health Statistics and Quality). 2015. "Behavioral Health Trends in the United States: Results from the 2014 National Survey on Drug Use and Health." Washington, DC: CBHSQ.

CDC (Centers for Disease Control and Prevention). 2015. *Reported Tuberculosis in the United States, 2014*. Atlanta, GA: CDC.

Chambers, Robert. 1983. *Rural Development: Putting the Last First*. London: Longman.

Chapman, Daniel P., Charles L. Whitfield, Vincent J. Felitti, Shanta R. Dube, Valerie J. Edwards, and Robert F. Anda. 2004. "Adverse Childhood Experiences and the Risk of Depressive Disorders in Adulthood." *Journal of Affective Disorders* 82: 217–25.

Chatterjee, Sudipto, Neerja Chowdhary, Sulochana Pednekar, Alex Cohen, Gracy Andrew, Ricardo Araya, Gregory Simon, Michael King, Shirley Telles, Helena Verdeli, et al. 2008. "Integrating Evidence-Based Treatments for Common Mental Disorders in Routine Primary Care: Feasibility and Acceptability of the MANAS Intervention in Goa, India." *World Psychiatry* 7 (1): 39–46.

Chokkanathan, Srinivasan. 2009. "Resources, Stressors and Psychological Distress among Older Adults in Chennai, India." *Social Science & Medicine* 68: 243–50.

Chopra, Mickey, Emmanuelle Daviaud, Robert Pattinson, Sharon Fonn, and Joy E. Lawn. 2009. "Saving the Lives of South Africa's Mothers, Babies, and Children: Can the Health System Deliver?" *Lancet* 374 (9692): 835–46.

Claassens, Mareli, Alliance Nikuze, Tawanda Chivese, Moleen Zunza, and Nulda Beyers. 2014. "Evidence to Inform South African Tuberculosis Policies (EVISAT) Project: A Systematic Review of the Epidemiology of and Programmatic Response to TB in People Living in Urban Informal Settlements in South Africa." The World Health Organization (WHO) commissioned the EVISAT project in support of the South Africa National Department of Health.

Closser, Svea. 2015. "Pakistan's Lady Health Worker Labor Movement and the Moral Economy of Heroism." *Annals of Anthropological Practice* 39 (1): 16–28.

Comaroff, Jean, and John Comaroff. 1991. *Of Revelation and Revolution: Christianity, Colonialism and Consciousness in South Africa*. Chicago: University of Chicago Press.

——. 1999. *Civil Society and the Political Imagination in Africa: Critical Perspectives*. Chicago: University of Chicago Press.

Cooper, Elizabeth. 2011. "Challenges and Opportunities in Inheritance Rights in Kenya." Policy Notes, Chronic Poverty Research Centre, London.

Coovadia, Hoosen, Rachel Jewkes, Peter Barron, David Sanders, and Diane McIntyre. 2009. "The Health and Health System of South Africa: Historical Roots of Current Public Health Challenges." *Lancet* 374 (9692): 817–34.

Crowther, Nigel J., and Shane A. Norris. 2012. "The Current Waist Circumference Cut Point Used for the Diagnosis of Metabolic Syndrome in Sub-Saharan African Women Is Not Appropriate." *PLoS ONE* 7 (11): e48883.

Danese, Andrea, Terrie E. Moffitt, HonaLee Harrington, Barry J. Milne, Guilherme Polanczyk, Carmine M. Pariante, Richie Poulton, and Avshalom Caspi. 2009. "Adverse Childhood Experiences and Adult Risk Factors for Age-Related Disease: Depression, Inflammation, and Clustering of Metabolic Risk Markers." *Archives of Pediatric and Adolescent Medicine* 163 (12): 1135–43.

Daniel, Mark, Kerin O'Dea, Kevin G Rowley, Robyn McDermott, and Shona Kelly. 1999. "Glycated Hemoglobin as an Indicator of Social Environmental Stress among Indigenous versus Westernized Populations." *Preventive Medicine* 29: 405–13.

Daniels, Mitchell E., Jr., Thomas E. Donilon, and Thomas J. Bollyky. 2014. "The Emerging Global Health Crisis: Noncommunicable Diseases in Low- and Middle-Income Countries." Council on Foreign Relations Press. New York, NY.

Das, Jishnu, Ranendra Kumar Das, and Veena Das. 2012. "The Mental Health Gender-Gap in Urban India: Patterns and Narratives." *Social Science & Medicine* 75 (9): 1660–72.

Das, Veena. 1997. "Language and Body: Transactions in the Construction of Pain." In *Social Suffering*, edited by Arthur Kleinman, Veena Das, and Margaret M. Lock, 67–92. Berkeley: University of California Press.

——. 2006. *Life and Words: Violence and the Descent into the Ordinary*. Berkeley: University of California Press.

——. 2008. "Violence, Gender, and Subjectivity." *Annual Review of Anthropology* 37: 283–99.

——. 2015. *Affliction: Health, Poverty, Disease*. New York: Fordham University Press.

Das Gupta, Monica. 1995. "Life Course Perspectives on Women's Autonomy and Health Outcomes." *American Anthropologist* 97 (3): 481–91.

Davis, Mike. 2006. *Planet of the Slums*. London: Verso.

De Genova, Nicholas, and Nathalie M. Peutz. 2010. *The Deportation Regime: Sovereignty, Space, and the Freedom of Movement*. Durham, NC: Duke University Press.

de Smedt, Johan Victor Adriaan de. 2011. "The Nubis of Kibera: A Social History of the Nubians and Kibera Slums." Doctoral thesis, Leiden University.

Denning, Paul, and Elizabeth Di Nenno. 2010. "Communities in Crisis: Is There a Generalized HIV Epidemic in Impoverished Urban Areas of the United States?" Centers for Disease Control and Prevention, National Center for HIV Viral Hepatitis STD and TB Prevention. Atlanta, GA: CDC.

Desjarlais, Robert. 2003. *Sensory Biographies: Lives and Deaths among Nepal's Yolmo Buddhists*. Berkeley: University of California Press.

Dong, Maxia, Robert F. Anda, Vincent J. Felitti, Shanta R. Dube, David F. Williamson, Theodore J. Thompson, Clifton M. Loo, and Wayne H. Giles. 2004a. "The Interrelatedness of Multiple Forms of Childhood Abuse, Neglect, and Household Dysfunction." *Child Abuse and Neglect* 28 (7): 771–84.

Dong, Maxia, Wayne H. Giles, Vincent J. Felitti, Shanta R. Dube, Janice E. Williams, Daniel P. Chapman, and Robert F. Anda. 2004b. "Insights into Causal Pathways for Ischemic Heart Disease: Adverse Childhood Experiences Study." *Circulation* 10: 1761–66.

Dunkle, Kristin L., Rachel K. Jewkes, Heather C. Brown, Mieko Yoshihama, Glenda E. Gray, James A. McIntyre, and Siobán D. Harlow. 2004. "Prevalence and Patterns of Gender-Based Violence and Revictimization among Women Attending Antenatal Clinics in Soweto, South Africa." *American Journal of Epidemiology* 160 (3): 230–39.

Dye, Christopher, Ties Boerma, David Evans, Anthony Harries, Christian Lienhardt, Joanne McManus, Tikki Pang, Robert Terry, Rony Zachariah. 2013. *Research for universal health coverage: World health report 2013.* World Health Organization. Geneva.

Edwards, Valerie J., George W. Holden, Vincent J. Felitti, and Robert F. Anda. 2003. "Experiencing Multiple Forms of Childhood Maltreatment and Adult Mental Health in Community Respondents: Results from the Adverse Childhood Experiences (ACE) Study." *American Journal of Psychiatry* 160 (8): 1453–60.

Ekdale, Brian. 2004. "Kibera's History." Unpublished Working Paper. University of Iowa. Iowa City, IA.

Ellison, George T. H., Thea de Wet, Carel B. Ijselmuiden, and Linda Richter. 1997. "Segregated Health Statistics Perpetuate Racial Stereotypes." *BMJ* 314: 1485.

Emeche, Uchenna. 2015. "Is a Strategy Focused on Super-Utilizers Equal to the Task of Health Care System Transformation? Yes." *Annals of Family Medicine* 13 (1): 6–7.

Epel, Elissa S., Bruce McEwen, Teresa Seeman, Karen Matthews, Grace Castellazzo, Kelly D. Brownell, Jennifer Bell, and Jeannette R. Ickovics. 2000. "Stress and Body Shape: Stress-Induced Cortisol Secretion Is Consistently Greater among Women with Central Fat." *Psychosomatic Medicine* 62: 623–32.

Epel, Elissa S., Rachel Lapidus, Bruce McEwen, and Kelly Brownell. 2001. "Stress May Add Bite to Appetite in Women: A Laboratory Study of Stress-Induced Cortisol and Eating Behavior." *Psychoneuroendocrinology* 26: 37–49.

Estroff, Sue. 1993. "Identity, Disability and Schizophrenia: The Problem of Chronicity." In *Knowledge, Power, and Practice: The Anthropology of Medicine and Everyday Life*, edited by Shirley Lindenbaum and Margaret M. Lock, 247–86. Berkeley: University of California Press.

Ewald, Paul W. 2008. "An Evolutionary Perspective on the Causes of Chronic Diseases: Atherosclerosis as an Illustration." In *Evolutionary Medicine and Health*, edited by Wendy R. Trevathan, E. O. Smith, and James J. McKenna. Pp. 245–270. Oxford, UK: Oxford University Press.

Farmer, Paul. 1996. "Social Inequalities and Emerging Infectious Diseases." *Emerging Infectious Diseases* 2 (4): 259–69.

——. 1997a. "On Suffering and Structural Violence: A View from Below." In *Social Suffering*, edited by Arthur Kleinman, Veena Das, and Margaret M. Lock. Pp 261–284. Berkeley: University of California Press.

——. 1997b. "Social Science and the New Tuberculosis." *Social Science & Medicine* 44 (3): 347–58.

——. 2001. *Infections and Inequalities: The Modern Plagues*. Berkeley: University of California.

——. 2004. *Pathologies of Power: Health, Human Rights, and the New War on the Poor*. Berkeley: University of California Press.

Farmer, Paul, Arthur Kleinman, Jim Yong Kim, and Matthew Basilico. 2013. *Reimagining Global Health: An Introduction*. Berkeley: University of California Press.

Farmer, Paul, Shirley Lindenbaum, and Mary-Jo Delvecchio Good. 1993. "Women, Poverty and AIDS: An Introduction." *Culture, Medicine & Psychiatry* 17 (4): 387–97.

Farr, Marcia. 2006. *Rancheros in Chicagoacán: Language and Identity in a Transnational Community*. Austin: University of Texas Press.

Fassin, Didier. 2002. "Embodied History: Uniqueness and Exemplarity of South African AIDS." *African Journal of AIDS Research* 1 (1): 63–68.

——. 2007. *When Bodies Remember: Experiences and Politics of AIDS in South Africa*. Berkeley: University of California Press.

——. 2009. "A Violence of History: Accounting for AIDS in Post-Apartheid South Africa." In *Global Health in Times of Violence*, edited by Barbara Rylko-Bauer, Linda Whiteford, and Paul Farmer, 113–36. Santa Fe, NM: School for Advanced Research Press.

Felitti, Vincent J., Robert F. Anda, Dale Nordenberg, David F. Williamson, Alison M. Spitz, Valarie Edwards, Mary P. Koss, and James S. Marks. 1998. "Relationship of Childhood Abuse and Household Dysfunction to Many of the Leading Causes of Death in Adults: The Adverse Childhood Experiences (ACE) Study." *American Journal of Preventive Medicine* 14 (4): 245–58.

Fernandes, Leela. 2004. "The Politics of Forgetting: Class Politics, State Power, and the Restructuring of Urban Space in India." *Urban Studies* 41 (12): 2415–30.

Ferreira, Mariana Leal, and Gretchen C. Lang, eds. 2006. *Indigenous Peoples and Diabetes: Community Empowerment and Wellness*. Durham, NC: Carolina Academic Press.

Ferzacca, Steve. 2000. "'Actually, I Don't Feel That Bad': Managing Diabetes and the Clinical Encounter." *Medical Anthropology Quarterly* 14 (1): 28–50.

——. 2012. "Diabetes and Culture." *Annual Review of Anthropology* 41 (1): 411–26.

Finkler, Kaja. 1994. *Women in Pain: Gender and Morbidity in Mexico*. Philadelphia: University of Philadelphia Press.

——. 1997. "Gender, Domestic Violence and Sickness in Mexico." *Social Science & Medicine* 45 (8): 1147–60.

——. 2000. "A Theory of Life's Lesions: A Contribution to Solving the Mystery of Why Women Get Sick more than Men." *Health Care for Women International* 21 (5): 433–55.

Fisher, Lawrence, Catherine A. Chesla, Marilyn M. Skaff, Catherine Gilliss, Joseph T. Mullan, Robert J. Bartz, Richard A. Kanter, and Claudia P. Lutz. 2000. "The Family and Disease Management in Hispanic and European-American Patients with Type 2 Diabetes." *Diabetes Care* 23 (3): 267–72.

Frenk, Julio, and Octavio Gómez-Dantés. 2017. "False Dichotomies in Global Health: The Need for Integrative Thinking." *Lancet* 389 (10069): 667–70.

Friedman, M. Reuel, Ron Stall, Anthony J. Silvestre, Chongyi Wei, Steve Shoptaw, Amy Herrick, Pamela J. Surkan, Linda Teplin, and Michael W. Plankey. 2015. "Effects of Syndemics on HIV Viral Load and Medication Adherence in the Multicentre AIDS Cohort Study." *AIDS* 29 (9): 1087–96.

Fuchsberger, Christian, Jason Flannick, Tanya M. Teslovich, Anubha Mahajan, Vineeta Agarwala, Kyle J. Gaulton, Clement Ma, et al. 2016. "The Genetic Architecture of Type 2 Diabetes." *Nature* 536 (7614): 41–47.

Gallaher, Courtney M., John M. Kerr, Mary Njenga, Nancy K. Karanja, and Antoinette M. G. A. WinklerPrins. 2013. "Urban Agriculture, Social Capital, and Food Security in the Kibera Slums of Nairobi, Kenya." *Agriculture and Human Values* 30 (3): 389–404.

Galtung, Johan. 1969. "Violence, Peace, and Peace Research." *Journal of Peace Research* 6 (3): 167–91.

García-Huidobro, Diego, Marcela Bittner, Paulina Brahm, and Klaus Puschel. 2011. "Family Intervention to Control Type 2 Diabetes: A Controlled Clinical Trial." *Family Practice* 28: 4–11.

Garro, Linda C. 2000. "Remembering What One Knows and the Construction of the Past: A Comparison of Cultural Knowledge of Cultural Consensus Theory and Cultural Schema Theory." *Ethos* 28 (3): 275–319.

Gawande, Atul. 2011. "The Hot Spotters: Can We Lower Medical Costs by Giving the Neediest Patients Better Care?" *The New Yorker* (January): 40–51.

Gilson, Lucy, and Anne Mills. 1995. "Health Sector Reforms in Sub-Saharan Africa: Lessons of the Last 10 Years." *Health Policy* 32: 215–43.

Gilson, Lucy, and Di McIntyre. 2005. "Removing User Fees for Primary Care in Africa: The Need for Careful Action." *BMJ* 331 (7519): 762–65.

Glaser, Clive. 2008. "Violent Crime in South Africa: Historical Perspectives." *South African Historical Journal* 60 (3): 334–52.

Goffman, Erving. 1959. *The Presentation of Self in Everyday Life*. New York. Anchor Books.

Golden, Sherita Hill, Hochang Benjamin Lee, Pamela J. Schreiner, Ana Diez Roux, Annette L. Fitzpatrick, Moyses Szklo, and Constantine Lyketsos. 2007. "Depression and Type 2 Diabetes Mellitus: The Multiethnic Study of Atherosclerosis." *Psychosomatic Medicine* 69 (6): 529–36.

Golden, Sherita Hill, Mariana Lazo, Mercedes Carnethon, and Patient Page. 2008. "Depressive Symptoms and Diabetes: Examining a Bidirectional Association Between Depression and Diabetes." *JAMA* 299 (23): 2751–59.

Gomero, Ada, Thomas McDade, Sharon Williams, Stacy Tessler Lindau. 2008. "Dried Blood Spot Measurement of Glycosylated Hemoglobin (HbA1c) in Wave 1 of the National Social Life, Health, and Aging Project, NORC and the University of Chicago. http://biomarkers.bsd.uchicago.edu/pdfs/TR-HbA1c.pdf.

Gomez-Oliver, F. Xavier, Margaret Thorogood, Philippe Bocquier, Paul Mee, Kathleen Kahn, Lisa Berkman, and Stephen Tollman. 2014. "Social Conditions and Disability Related to the Mortality of Older People in Rural South Africa." *International Journal of Epidemiology* 43 (5): 1531–41.

Good, Byron. 1994. *Medicine, Rationality, and Experience: An Anthropological Perspective*. Cambridge, UK: Cambridge University Press.

Goudge, Jane, Lucy Gilson, Steven Russell, Tebogo Gumede, and Anne Mills. 2009. "Affordability, Availability and Acceptability Barriers to Health Care for the Chronically Ill: Longitudinal Case Studies from South Africa." *BMC Health Services Research* 18: 1–18.

Gradidge, Philippe Jean-Luc, Shane A. Norris, Nicole G. Jaff, and Nigel J. Crowther. 2016. "Metabolic and Body Composition Risk Factors Associated with Metabolic Syndrome in a Cohort of Women with a High Prevalence of Cardiometabolic Disease." *PLoS ONE* 11 (9): e0162247.

Green, Linda. 1999. *Fear as a Way of Life: Mayan Widows in Rural Guatemala*. New York: Columbia University Press.

Gregg, Edward W., Xiaohui Zhuo, Yiling J. Cheng, Ann L. Albright, K. M. Venkat Narayan, and Theodore J. Thompson. 2014. "Trends in Lifetime Risk and Years of Life Lost Due to Diabetes in the USA, 1985–2011: A Modelling Study." *Lancet Diabetes & Endocrinology* 2 (11): 867–74.

Guariguata, Leonor, David R. Whiting, Ian R. Hambleton, Jessica Beagley, Ute Linnenkamp, and Jonathan E. Shaw. 2014. "Global Estimates of Diabetes Prevalence for 2013 and Projections for 2035." *Diabetes Research and Clinical Practice* 103 (2): 137–49.

Guerra, F. B. Del, J. L. I. Fonseca, V. M. Figueiredo, E. B. Ziff, and E. Castelon Konkiewitz. 2013. "Human Immunodeficiency Virus–Associated Depression: Contributions of Immuno-Inflammatory, Monoaminergic, Neurodegenerative, and Neurotrophic Pathways." *Journal of NeuroVirology* 19 (4): 314–27.

Gunnar, Megan R. 2000. "Early Adversity and the Development of Stress Reactivity and Regulation." In *The Effects of Early Adversity on Neurobehavioral Development: The Minnesota Symposium on Child Psychology*, vol. 31, edited by C. A. Nelson, 163–200. Mahwah, NJ: Lawrence Erlbuam Associates Publishers.

Gutmann, Matthew. 1999. "Ethnicity, Alcohol, and Acculturation." *Social Science & Medicine* 48: 173–84.

Hajjebrahimi, B., A. Kiamanesh, A. A. Asgharnejad Farid, and G. Asadikaram. 2016. "Type 2 Diabetes and Mental Disorders; a Plausible Link with Inflammation." *Cellular and Molecular Biology* 62 (13): 71–77.

Hall, H. Irene, Qian An, Tian Tang, Ruiguang Song, Mi Chen, Timothy Green, Jian Kang, and Centers for Disease Control and Prevention (CDC). 2015. "Prevalence of Diagnosed and Undiagnosed HIV Infection—United States, 2008–2012." *Morbidity and Mortality Weekly Report* 64 (24): 657–62.

Hansen, Thomas Blom. 2011. "From Culture to Barbed Wire: On Houses and Walls in South Africa." *Texas International Law Journal* 46 (1949): 345–53.

Hardin, Jessica. 2015. "'Healing is a Done Deal': Temporality and Metabolic Healing Among Evangelical Christians in Samoa." *Medical Anthropology* 35 (2), 105–18.

—— 2018. *Faith and the Pursuit of Health: Cardiometabolic Disorders in Samoa*. New Brunswick: Rutgers University Press.

Health and Development Africa. 2012. *Global Aids Response Republic of South Africa*. Johannesburg, South Africa: UNGASS.

Heilemann, MarySue V., Felix Salvador Kury, and Kathryn A. Lee. 2005. "Trauma and Posttraumatic Stress Disorder Symptoms among Low Income Women of Mexican Descent in the United States." *The Journal of Nervous and Mental Disease* 193 (10): 665–72.

Hercot, David, Bruno Meessen, Valery Ridde, and Lucy Gilson. 2011. "Removing User Fees for Health Services in Low-Income Countries: A Multi-Country Review Framework for Assessing the Process of Policy Change." *Health Policy and Planning* 26: ii5–ii15.

Herman, Allen, Dan Stein, Soraya Seedat, Steven G. Heeringa, Hashim Moomal, and David R. Williams. 2009. "The South African Stress and Health (SASH) Study: 12- Month and Lifetime Prevalence of Common Mental Disorders." *South African Medical Journal* 99 (5): 339–44.

Herrick, Amy L., Sin How Lim, Michael W. Plankey, Joan S. Chmiel, Thomas T. Guadamuz, Uyen Kao, Steven Shoptaw, Adam Carrico, David Ostrow, and Ron Stall. 2013. "Adversity and Syndemic Production among Men Participating in the Multicenter AIDS Cohort Study: A Life-Course Approach." *American Journal of Public Health* 103 (1): 79–85.

Herrick, Clare. 2017. "When Places Come First: Suffering, Archetypal Space and the Problematic Production of Global Health." *Transactions of the Institute of British Geographers* 42 (4): 530–43.

Himmelgreen, David, Nancy Romero-Daza, David Turkon, Sharon Watson, Ipolto Okello-Uma, and Daniel Sellen. 2009. "Addressing the HIV/AIDS-Food Insecurity Syndemic in Sub-Saharan Africa." *African Journal of AIDS Research* 8 (4): 401–12.

Hirsch, Jennifer. 2003. *A Courtship after Marriage: Sexuality and Love in Mexican Transnational Families.* Berkeley: University of California Press.

Holmes, Seth. 2013. *Fresh Fruits, Broken Bodies: Migrant Farmworkers in the United States.* Berkeley: University of California Press.

Holt, Richard I. G., Mary De Groot, and Sherita Hill Golden. 2014. "Diabetes and Depression." *Current Diabetes Report* 14: 491.

Hoogeveen, Johannes G., and Berk Özler. 2005. "Not Separate, Not Equal: Poverty and Inequality in Post-Apartheid South Africa." Working Paper No. 739, William Davidson Institute, University of Michigan, Ann Arbor.

Huchzermeyer, Marie. 2008. "Slum Upgrading in Nairobi within the Housing and Basic Services Market: A Housing Rights Concern." *Journal of Asian and African Studies* 43 (1): 19–39.

Hulzebosch, Annelieke, Steven van de Vijver, Thaddaeus Egondi, Samuel O. Oti, and Catherine Kyobutungi. 2015. "Profile of People with Hypertension in Nairobi's Slums: A Descriptive Study." *Globalization and Health* 11 (1): 26.

Hunt, Linda M. 1998. "Moral Reasoning and the Meaning of Cancer: Causal Explanations of Oncologists and Patients in Southern Mexico." *Medical Anthropology Quarterly* 12 (3): 298–318.

Hunt, Linda M., C. H. Browner, and Brigitte Jordan. 1990. "Hypoglycemia: Portrait of an Illness Construct in Everyday Use." *Medical Anthropology Quarterly* 4 (2): 191–210.

Hunt, Linda M., Miguel A. Valenzuela, and Jacqueline A. Pugh. 1998. "Porque Me Tocó a Mi? Mexican American Diabetes Patients' Causal Stories and Their Relationship to Treatment Behaviors." *Social Science & Medicine* 46 (8): 959–69.

Hunt, Linda M., Suzanne Schneider, and Brendon Comer. 2004. "Should 'Acculturation' Be a Variable in Health Research? A Critical Review of Research on US Hispanics." *Social Science & Medicine* 59 (5): 973–86.

IDF (International Diabetes Federation). 2013. *IDF Diabetes Atlas*. Brussels, Belgium: IDF. 6th ed.

———. 2015. *IDF Diabetes Atlas*. Brussels, Belgium: IDF. 7th ed.

Inhorn, Marcia C. 2006. "Defining Women's Health: A Dozen Messages from More than 150 Ethnographies." *Medical Anthropology Quarterly* 20 (3): 345–78.

International Union against Tuberculosis and Lung Disease (The Union). 2012. *The Union: Health Solutions for the Poor*. Paris: The Union. http://www.theunion.org.

Jan, Stephen, Tracey Lea Laba, Beverley M. Essue, Adrian Gheorghe, Janani Muhunthan, Michael Engelgau, Ajay Mahal, et al. 2018. "Action to Address the Household Economic Burden of Non-Communicable Diseases." *Lancet* 6736 (18): 1–12.

Jenkins, J. (2015). *Extraordinary Conditions: Culture and Experience in Mental Illness*. Berkeley: University of California Press.

Joireman, Sandra, and Rachel Sweet Vanderpoel. 2008. "In Search of Order: Property Rights Enforcement in Kibera Settlement, Kenya." Working paper. August 13. SSRN.

Joshi, Rohina, Mohammed Alim, Andre Pascal Kengne, Stephen Jan, Pallab K. Maulik, David Peiris, and Anushka A. Patel. 2014. "Task Shifting for Non-Communicable Disease Management in Low and Middle Income Countries—A Systematic Review." *PLoS ONE* 9 (8): e103754.

Kadam, Swapna S., B. S. Payghan, R. Mayuri Reddy, and Kumara Swamy. 2014. "Role of Social Determinants in Glycemic Control of Type 2 Diabetic Subjects." *International Research Journal of Medical Sciences* 2 (4): 2–6.

Kaiser, Bonnie, Emily E. Haroz, Brandon A. Kohrt, Paul A. Bolton, Judith K. Bass, and Devon E. Hinton. 2015. "'Thinking Too Much': A Systematic Review of a Common Idiom of Distress." *Social Science & Medicine* 147: 170–83.

Kaiser, Paulina, Amy H. Auchincloss, Kari Moore, Brisa N. Sánchez, Veronica Berrocal, Norrina Allen, and Ana V. Diez. 2016. "Associations of Neighborhood Socioeconomic and Racial/Ethnic Characteristics with Changes in Survey-Based Neighborhood Quality, 2000–2011." *Health & Place* 42: 30–36.

Kakuma, Ritsuko, Harry Minas, Nadja Van Ginneken, Mario R. Dal Poz, Keshav Desiraju, Jodi E. Morris, Shekhar Saxena, and Richard M. Scheffler. 2011. "Human Resources for Mental Health Care: Current Situation and Strategies for Action." *Lancet* 378 (9803): 1654–63.

Kalofonos, Ippolytos. 2014. "'All They Do Is Pray': Community Labour and the Narrowing of 'Care' during Mozambique's HIV Scale-Up." *Global Public Health* 9 (1–2): 7–24.

Kant, Lalit. 2003. "Diabetes Mellitus-Tuberculosis: The Brewing Double Trouble." *Indian Journal of Tuberculosis* 50 (4): 83–84.

Karim, Salim S. Abdool, Gavin J. Churchyard, Quarraisha Abdool Karim, and Stephen D. Lawn. 2009. "HIV Infection and Tuberculosis in South Africa: An Urgent Need to Escalate the Public Health Response." *Lancet* 374: 921–33.

Kenworthy, Nora J. 2017. *Mistreated: The Political Consequences of the Fight against AIDS in Lesotho*. Nashville, TN: Vanderbilt University Press.

Kenworthy, Nora, Matthew Thomann, and Richard Parker. 2017. "From a Global Crisis to the 'End of AIDS': New Epidemics of Signification." *Global Public Health* 13 (8): 960–71.

Kenworthy, Nora, and Richard Parker. 2014. "Introduction: HIV Scale-Up and the Politics of Global Health." *Global Public Health* 9 (1–2): 1–6.

Kessler, Ronald C., and Evelyn J. Bromet. 2013. "The Epidemiology of Depression across Cultures." *Annual Review of Public Health* 34: 119–38.

Kessler, Ronald C., Sergio Aguilar-Gaxiola, Jordi Alonso, Somnath Chatterji, Sing Lee, Johan Ormel, T. Bedirham Üstün, and Phillip S. Wang. 2009. "The Global Burden of Mental Disorders: An Update from the WHO World Mental Health (WMH) Surveys." *Epidemiologia e Psichiatria Sociale* 18 (1): 23–33.

Kidder, Alice, Gene Kwan, Corrado Cancedda, and Gene Bukhman. 2011. *Chronic Care Integration for Endemic Non-Communicable Diseases: Rwanda Edition*. Boston, MA: Partners in Health.

Kien, Vu Duy, Hoang Van Minh, Kim Bao Giang, Amy Dao, Le Thanh Tuan, and Nawi Ng. 2016. "Socioeconomic Inequalities in Catastrophic Health Expenditure and Impoverishment Associated with Non-Communicable Diseases in Urban Hanoi, Vietnam." *International Journal for Equity in Health* 15 (1): 169.

Kimuna, Sitawa R., and Yanyi K. Kjamba. 2008. "Gender Based Violence: Correlates of Physical and Sexual Wife Abuse in Kenya." *Journal of Family Violence* 23 (5): 333–42.

Kirmayer, Laurence. J. 2012. "Rethinking Cultural Competence." *Transcultural Psychiatry*, 49: 149–164.

Kirmayer, Laurence J. 2006. "Beyond the 'New Cross-Cultural Psychiatry': Cultural Biology, Discursive Psychology and the Ironies of Globalization." *Transcultural Psychiatry* 43: 126–44.

Kirmayer, Laurence J., Robert Lemelson, and Mark Barad. 2007. *Understanding Trauma: Integrating Biological, Clinical, and Cultural Perspectives*. Cambridge, UK: Cambridge University Press.

Kleinman, Arthur. 1980. *Patients and Healers in the Context of Culture: An Exploration of the Borderland Between Anthropology, Medicine, and Psychiatry*. Berkeley: University of California Press.

———. 1986. *Social Origins of Distress and Disease: Depression, Neurasthenia, and Pain in Modern China*. New Haven, CT: Yale University Press.

———. 1988. *The Illness Narratives: Suffering, Healing, and the Human Condition*. New York: Basic Books.

———. 1995. *Writing at the Margin: Discourse between Anthropology and Medicine*. Berkeley: University of California Press.

———. 1999. "Experience and Its Moral Modes: Culture, Human Conditions and Disorder." In *The Tanner Lectures on Human Values*, 357–420. Stanford, CA: Stanford University Press.

———. 2010. "Four Social Theories for Global Health." *Lancet* 375 (9725): 1518–19.

Kleinman, Arthur, Veena Das, and Margaret M. Lock. 1997. *Social Suffering*. Berkeley: University of California Press.

Knol, Mirjam Judith, Jos W. R. Twisk, Aartjan T. F. Beekman, Robert J. Heine, Frank J. Snoek, and Francois Pouwer. 2006. "Depression as a Risk Factor for the Onset of Type 2 Diabetes Mellitus: A Meta-Analysis." *Diabetologia* 49 (5): 837–45.

Knut, Lönnroth, Gojka Roglic, and Anthony D. Harries. 2014. "Improving Tuberculosis Prevention and Care through Addressing the Global Diabetes Epidemic: From Evidence to Policy and Practice." *Lancet Diabetes & Endocrinology* 2 (9): 730–39.

Kohrt, Brandon A., Andrew Rasmussen, Bonnie N. Kaiser, Emily E. Haroz, Sujen M. Maharjan, Byamah B. Mutamba, Joop T. V. M. De Jong, and Devon E. Hinton. 2014. "Cultural Concepts of Distress and Psychiatric Disorders: Literature Review and Research Recommendations for Global Mental Health Epidemiology." *International Journal of Epidemiology* 43 (2): 365–406.

Krieger, Nancy. 1994. "Epidemiology and the Web of Causation: Has Anyone Seen the Spider?" *Social Science & Medicine* 39 (7): 887–903.

———. 2001. "Theories for Social Epidemiology in the 21st Century: An Ecosocial Perspective." *International Journal of Epidemiology* 30: 668–77.

Krieger, Nancy, and George Davey Smith. 2004. "'Bodies Count,' and Body Counts: Social Epidemiology and Embodying Inequality." *Epidemiologic Reviews* 26: 92–103.

Kuzawa, Christopher W. 2008. "The Developmental Origins of Adult Health: Intergenerational Inertia in Adaptation and Disease." In *Evolutionary Medicine and Health*, edited by Wenda R. Trevathan, E. O. Smith, and James J. McKenna, 325–49. Oxford, UK: Oxford University Press.

Kuzawa, Christopher W., and Elizabeth A. Quinn. 2009. "Developmental Origins of Adult Function and Health: Evolutionary Hypotheses." *Annual Review of Anthropology* 38 (1): 131–47.

Kuzawa, Christopher W., and Elizabeth Sweet. 2009. "Epigenetics and the Embodiment of Race: Developmental Origins of US Racial Disparities in Cardiovascular Health." *American Journal of Human Biology* 21 (1): 2–15.

Lancet Diabetes & Endocrinology. 2014. "Diabetes and Tuberculosis—A Wake Up Call." *Lancet Diabetes & Endocrinology* 2 (9): 677.

Lang, Tim, and Michael Heasman. 2015. *Food Wars: The Global Battle for Mouths, Minds, and Markets*. New York: Routledge.

Lawn, Stephen D, Linda-Gail Bekker, Keren Middelkoop, Landon Myer, and Robin Wood. 2006. "Impact of HIV Infection on the Epidemiology of Tuberculosis in a Peri-Urban Community in South Africa: The Need for Age-Specific Interventions." *Clinical Infectious Diseases: An Official Publication of the Infectious Diseases Society of America* 42 (7): 1040–47.

Le Marcis, Frédéric. 2012. "Struggling with AIDS in South Africa: The Space of the Everyday as a Field of Recognition." *Medical Anthropology Quarterly* 26 (4): 486–502.

Lee, Chioun, Vera Tsenkova, and Deborah Carr. 2012. "Childhood Trauma and Metabolic Syndrome in Men and Women." *Social Science & Medicine* 29 (6): 997–1003.

Leone, Tiziana, Ernestina Coast, Shilpa Narayanan, and Ama De-Graft Aikins. 2012. "Diabetes and Depression Comorbidity and Socio-Economic Status in Low and Middle Income Countries (LMICs): A Mapping of the Evidence." *Globalization and Health* 8: 39.

Lévi-Strauss, Claude. 1969. *The Elementary Structures of Kinship*. New York: Beacon Press.

Lewis, Patrick R. B. 1966. *A "City" within a City: The Creation of Soweto*. Johannesburg, South Africa: University of the Witwatersrand.

Lewis, Sara E. 2013. "Trauma and the Making of Flexible Minds in the Tibetan Exile Community." *Ethos* 41 (3): 313–36.

——. 2018. "Resilience, Agency, and Everyday Lojong in the Tibetan Diaspora." *Contemporary Buddhism: An Interdisciplinary Journal*. 1–20, epub May 29.

Lieberman, Leslie. 2003. "Dietary, Evolutionary, and Modernizing Influences on the Prevalence of Type 2 Diabetes." *Annual Review of Nutrition* 23: 345–77.

——. 2008. "Diabesity and Darwinian Medicine: The Evolution of an Epidemic." In *Evolutionary Medicine and Health*, edited by Wenda R. Trevathan, E. O. Smith, and James J. McKenna, 72–95. Oxford, UK: Oxford University Press.

Lindenbaum, Shirley. 1979. *Kuru Sorcery: Disease and Danger in the New Guinea Highlands*. Palo Alto, CA: Mayfield.

Link, Bruce G., and Jo Phelan. 1995. "Social Conditions as Fundamental Causes of Disease." *Journal of Health and Social Behavior* 35: 80–94.

Lock, Margaret. 1993. *Encounters with Aging: Mythologies of Menopause in Japan and North America*. Berkeley: University of California Press.

——. 2001. "The Tempering of Medical Anthropology: Troubling Natural Categories." *Medical Anthropology Quarterly* 15 (4): 478–92.

Lohrmann, Graham M., B. Botha, Avy Violari, and Glenda E. Gray. 2012. "HIV and the Urban Homeless in Johannesburg." *Southern African Journal of HIV Medicine* 13 (4): 2010–13.

Lovallo, William R., and Terrie L. Thomas. 2000. "Stress Hormones in Psychophysiological Research: Emotional, Behavioral, and Cognitive Implications." In *Handbook of Psychophysiology*, edited by John Cacciopo, Louis Tassinary, and Gary Bernston, 342–67. Cambridge, UK: Cambridge University Press. 2nd ed.

Lown, E. Anne, and William A. Vega. 2001. "Prevalence and Predictors of Physical Partner Abuse among Mexican American Women." *American Journal of Public Health* 91 (3): 441–45.

Ludwig, Jens, Lisa Sanbonmatsu, Lisa Gennetian, Emma Adam, Greg J. Duncan, Lawrence F. Katz, Ronald C. Kessler, et al. 2011. "Neighborhoods, Obesity, and Diabetes—A Randomized Social Experiment." *New England Journal of Medicine* 365 (16): 1509–19.

Lund, Crick, Alison Breen, Alan J. Flisher, Ritsuko Kakuma, Joanne Corrigall, John A. Joska, Leslie Swartz, and Vikram Patel. 2010. "Poverty and Common Mental Disorders in Low and Middle Income Countries: A Systematic Review." *Social Science & Medicine* 71 (3): 517–28.

Lund, Crick, Mark Tomlinson, Mary de Silva, Abebaw Fekadu, Rahul Shidhaye, Mark Jordans, Inge Petersen, et al. 2012. "PRIME: A Programme to Reduce the Treatment Gap for Mental Disorders in Five Low- and Middle-Income Countries." *PLoS Medicine* 9 (12): e1001359.

Lund, Crick, Mark Tomlinson, and Vikram Patel. 2015. "Integration of Mental Health into Primary Care in Low- and Middle-Income Countries: The PRIME Mental Healthcare Plans." *British Journal of Psychiatry* 208 (Suppl. 56): s1–3.

Lutfey, Karen, and Jeremy Freese. 2005. "Toward Some Fundamentals of Fundamental Causality: Socioeconomic Status and Health in the Routine Clinic Visit for Diabetes." *American Journal of Sociology* 110 (5): 1326–72.

Madise, Nyovani, Abdhalah K. Ziraba, Joseph Inungu, Samoel A. Khamadi, Alex Ezeh, Eliya M. Zulu, John Kebaso, Vincent Okoth, and Matilu Mwau. 2012. "Are Slum Dwellers at Heightened Risk of HIV Infection than Other Urban Residents? Evidence from Population-Based HIV Prevalence Surveys in Kenya." *Health & Place* 18 (5): 1144–52.

Maes, Kenneth. 2015. "Community Health Workers and Social Change." *Annals of Anthropological Practice* 39 (1): 1–15.

———. 2016. *The Lives of Community Health Workers: Local Labor and Global Health in Urban Ethiopia.* New York: Routledge.

Maes, Kenneth, Svea Closser, Ethan Vorel, and Yihenew Tesfaye. 2015a. "A Women's Development Army: Narratives of Community Health Worker Investment and Empowerment in Rural Ethiopia." *Studies in Comparative International Development* 50 (4): 455–78.

———. 2015b. "Using Community Health Workers." *Annals of Anthropological Practice* 39 (1): 42–57.

Magadi, Monica. 2013. "The Disproportionate High Risk of HIV Infection among the Urban Poor in Sub-Saharan Africa." *AIDS and Behavior* 17 (5): 1645–54.

Makinen, Marty, Hugh Waters, M. Rauch, Naila Almagambetova, Ricardo Bitran, Lucy Gilson, Di Mcintyre, S. Pannarunothai, Amy L. Prieto, Gloria Ubilla, and Sujata Ram. 2000. "Inequalities in Health Care Use and Expenditures: Empirical Data from Eight Developing Countries and Countries in Transition." *Bulletin of the World Health Organization* 78 (1): 55–65.

Mamlin, Joseph, Sylvester Kimaiyo, Stephen Lewis, Hannah Tadayo, Fanice Komen Jerop, Catherine Gichunge, Tomeka Petersen, Yuehwern Yih, Paula Braitstein, and Robert Einterz. 2009. "Integrating Nutrition Support for Food-Insecure Patients and Their Dependents into an HIV Care and Treatment Program in Western Kenya." *American Journal of Public Health* 99 (2): 215–21.

Manderson, Lenore, and Carolyn Smith-Morris. 2010. *Chronic Conditions, Fluid States: Chronicity and the Anthropology of Illness.* New Brunswick, NJ: Rutgers University Press.

Mankekar, Punima. 1998. "Entangled Spaces of Modernity: The Viewing Family, the Consuming Nation, and Television in India." *Visual Anthropology Review* 14 (2): 32–45.

Marmot, Michael. 2005. "Public Health Social Determinants of Health Inequalities." *Lancet* 365: 1099–104.

———. 2007. "Achieving Health Equity: From Root Causes to Fair Outcomes." *Lancet* 370 (9593): 1153–63.

Marmot, Michael, Geoffrey Rose, Michael Shipley, and Patrick J. Hamilton. 1978. "Employment Grade and Coronary Heart Disease in British Civil Servants." *Journal of Epidemiology and Community Health* 32: 244–49.

Marmot, Michael, and Michael E. McDowall. 1986. "Mortality Decline and Widening Social Inequalities." *Lancet* 2 (8501): 274–76.

Marrow, Jocelyn. 2013. "Feminine Power or Feminine Weakness? North Indian Girls' Struggles with Aspirations, Agency, and Psychosomatic Illness." *American Ethnologist* 40 (2): 347–61.

Marshall, Mac. 2014. *Drinking Smoke: The Tobacco Syndemic in Oceania.* Honolulu: University of Hawaii Press.

Mattingly, Cheryl. 1998. *Healing Dramas and Clinical Plots: The Narrative Structure of Experience.* Cambridge, UK: Cambridge University Press.

Mattingly, Cheryl, and Linda Garro. 2000. *Narrative and the Cultural Construction of Illness and Healing.* Berkeley: University of California Press.

Mayosi, Bongani M., Alan J. Flisher, Umesh G. Lalloo, Freddy Sitas, Stephen M. Tollman, and Debbie Bradshaw. 2009. "The Burden of Non-Communicable Diseases in South Africa." *Lancet* 374 (9693): 934–47.

Mayosi, Bongani M., Joy E. Lawn, Ashley Van Niekerk, Debbie Bradshaw, Salim S. Abdool Karim, Hoosen M. Coovadia, and Lancet South Africa Team. 2012. "Health in South Africa: Changes and Challenges since 2009." *Lancet* 6736 (12): 5–19.

McDade, Thomas W., Louise C. Hawkley, and John T. Cacioppo. 2006. "Psychosocial and Behavioral Predictors of Inflammation in Middle-Aged and Older Adults: The Chicago Health, Aging, and Social Relations Study." *Psychosomatic Medicine* 68: 376–81.

McEwen, Bruce, and Teresa Seeman. 1999. "Protective and Damaging Effects of Mediators of Stress Elaborating and Testing the Concepts of Allostasis and Allostatic Load." *Annals of the New York Academy of Sciences* 896: 30–47.

McGarvey, Stephen T. 2009. "Interdisciplinary Translational Research in Anthropology, Nutrition, and Public Health." *Annual Review of Anthropology* 38: 233–49.

McGarvey, Stephen T., Jim R. Bindon, Douglas E. Crews, and Diana E. Schendel. 1989. "Modernization and Adiposity: Causes and Consequences." In *Human Population Biology*, edited by Michael Little and Jere D. Haas, 263–80. London: Oxford University Press.

McGuire, Megan, Jihane Ben Farhat, Gaelle Pedrono, Elisabeth Szumilin, Annette Heinzelmann, Yamikani Ntakwile Chinyumba, Sylvie Goossens, Simon Makombe, and Mar Pujades-Rodríguez. 2013. "Task-Sharing of HIV Care and ART Initiation: Evaluation of a Mixed-Care Non-Physician Provider Model for ART Delivery in Rural Malawi." *PLoS ONE* 8 (9): 1–10.

Menary, Richard. 2008. "Embodied Narratives." *Journal of Consciousness Studies* 15 (6): 63–84.

Mendenhall, Emily. 2012. *Syndemic Suffering: Social Distress, Depression, and Diabetes among Mexican Immigrant Women.* New York, NY: Routledge.

———. 2015a. "Beyond Comorbidity: A Critical Perspective of Syndemic Depression and Diabetes in Cross-Cultural Contexts." *Medical Anthropology Quarterly* 30 (4): 462–78.

———. 2015b. "Syndemic Suffering in Soweto: Violence and Inequality at the Nexus of Health Transition in South Africa." *Annals of Anthropological Practice* 38 (2): 302–18.

———. 2017. "Syndemics: A New Path for Global Health Research." *Lancet* 389: 889–91.

Mendenhall, Emily, Alicia Fernandez, Nancy Adler, and Elizabeth A. Jacobs. 2012a. "Susto, Coraje, and Abuse: Depression and Beliefs about Diabetes." *Culture, Medicine and Psychiatry* 36 (3): 480–92.

Mendenhall, Emily, Brandon Kohrt, Shane Norris, David Ndetei, and Dorairaj Prabhakaran. 2017. "Non-Communicable Disease Syndemics: Poverty, Depression, and Diabetes among the Urban Poor." *Lancet* 389: 951–63.

Mendenhall, Emily, Gregory Barnabas Omondi, Edna Bosire, Isaiah Gitonga, Abednego Musau, David Ndetei, and Victoria Mutiso. 2015. "Stress, Diabetes, and Infection: Syndemic Suffering in an Urban Public Hospital Clinic in Kenya." *Social Science & Medicine* 146: 11–20.

Mendenhall, Emily, Linda M. Richter, Alan Stein, and Shane A. Norris. 2013. "Psychological and Physical Co-Morbidity among Urban South African Women." *PLoS One* 8 (10): e78803.

Mendenhall, Emily, Rebecca A. Seligman, Alicia Fernandez, and Elizabeth A. Jacobs. 2010. "Speaking through Diabetes: Rethinking the Significance of Lay Discourses on Diabetes." *Medical Anthropology Quarterly* 24 (2): 220–39.

Mendenhall, Emily, Rebecca Rinehart, Christine W. Musyimi, Edna Bosire, David M. Ndetei, and Victoria Mutiso. 2019. "An Ethnopsychology of Idioms of Distress in Urban Kenya." *Transcultural Psychiatry*. epub Jan. 23.

Mendenhall, Emily, Roopa Shivashankar, Nikhil Tandon, Mohammed K. Ali, K. M. Venkat Narayan, and Dorairaj Prabhakaran. 2012b. "Stress and Diabetes in Socioeconomic Context: A Qualitative Study of Urban Indians." *Social Science & Medicine* 75 (12): 2522–29.

Mendenhall, Emily, and Shane A. Norris. 2015a. "Diabetes Care among Urban Women in Soweto, South Africa: A Qualitative Study." *BMC Public Health* 15 (1): 1300.

——. 2015b. "When HIV Is Ordinary and Diabetes New: Remaking Suffering in a South African Township." *Global Public Health* 10 (4): 449–62.

Mendenhall, Emily, Shane A. Norris, Rahul Shidhaye, and Dorairaj Prabhakaran. 2014. "Depression and Type 2 Diabetes in Low- and Middle-Income Countries: A Systematic Review." *Diabetes Research and Clinical Practice* 103 (2): 276–85.

Meyer, Pamela A., Paula W. Yoon, and Rachel B. Kaufmann. 2013. "Introduction: CDC Health Disparities and Inequalities Report—United States, 2013 Surveillance Summaries." *Morbidity and Mortality Weekly Report* 62 (Suppl. 3): 3–5.

Mezuk, Briana, Åsa Chaikiat, Xinjun Li, Jan Sundquist, Kenneth S. Kendler, and Kristina Sundquist. 2013. "Depression, Neighborhood Deprivation and Risk of Type 2 Diabetes." *Health & Place* 23: 63–69.

Miles, Jeremy N. V., Grant N. Marshall, and Terry L. Schell. 2008. "Spanish and English Versions of the PTSD Checklist—Civilian Version: Testing for Differential Item Functioning." *Journal of Traumatic Stress* 21(4): 369–76.

Ministry of Health and Family Welfare. 2006. *National Family Health Survey (NHFS3), 2005–06*. Delhi: Ministry of Health and Family Welfare.

Ministry of Health & Family Welfare Urban Health Division. 2006. *Health of the Urban Poor in India: Key Results from the National Family Health Survey, 2005–06*. Delhi: Ministry of Health & Family Welfare.

Mintz, Sidney. 1985. *Sweetness and Power: The Place of Sugar in Modern History*. New York: Penguin Books.

Misra, A Pandey, R. M. Devi, J. R. Sharma, R. Vikram, N. K. Khanna, N. 2001. "High Prevalence of Diabetes, Obesity and Dyslipidaemia in Urban Slum Population in

Northern India." *International Journal of Obesity Related Metabolic Disorders* 25 (11): 1722–29.

Mohan, V., Sreedharan Sandeep, Raj Deepa, Bhaskar Shah, and Cherian Varghese. 2007. "Epidemiology of Type 2 Diabetes: Indian Scenario." *The Indian Journal of Medical Research* 125: 217–30.

Mol, Annemarie, and John Law. 2004. "Embodied Action, Enacted Bodies: The Example of Hypoglycaemia." *Body & Society* 10 (2–3): 43–62.

Monahan, Patrick O., Enbal Shacham, Michael Reece, Kurt Kroenke, Willis Owino Ong'Or, Otieno Omollo, Violet Naanyu Yebei, and Claris Ojwang. 2009. "Validity/Reliability of PHQ-9 and PHQ-2 Depression Scales among Adults Living with HIV/AIDS in Western Kenya." *Journal of General Internal Medicine* 24 (2): 189–97.

Monteiro, Carlos Augusto, Jean-Claude Moubarac, Geoffrey Cannon, Shu Wen Ng, and Barry Popkin. 2013. "Ultra-Processed Products Are Becoming Dominant in the Global Food System." *Obesity Reviews* 14 (S2): 21–28.

Montoya, Michael J. 2007. "Bioethnic Conscription: Genes, Race, and Mexicana/o Ethnicity in Diabetes Research." *Cultural Anthropology* 22 (1): 94–128.

——. 2011. *Making the Mexican Diabetic: Race, Science, and the Genetics of Inequality*. Berkeley: University of California Press.

Moran-Thomas, Amy. 2012. "Metabola: Chronic Life in Belize." PhD diss., Anthropology Department, Princeton University.

Moulton, Calum D., John C. Pickup, and Khalida Ismail. 2015. "The Link between Depression and Diabetes: The Search for Shared Mechanisms." *Lancet* 3: 461–71.

Mugisha, Joseph O., Enid J. Schatz, Madeleine Randell, Monica Kuteesa, Paul Kowal, Joel Negin, and Janet Seeley. 2016. "Chronic Disease, Risk Factors and Disability in Adults Aged 50 and above Living with and without HIV: Findings from the Wellbeing of Older People Study in Uganda." *Global Health Action* 9: 31098.

Mullings, Leith. 2005. "Resistance and Resilience: The Sojourner Syndrome and the Social Context of Reproduction in Central Harlem." *Transforming Anthropology* 13 (2): 79–91.

Musselman, Dominique L., Ephi Betan, Hannah Larsen, and Lawrence S. Phillips. 2003. "Relationship of Depression to Diabetes Types 1 and 2: Epidemiology, Biology, and Treatment." *Biological Psychiatry* 54 (3): 317–29.

Mutahi, Patrick. 2011. "Between Illegality and Legality: (In)Security, Crime, and Gangs in Nairobi Informal Settlements." *South Africa Crime Quarterly* 37: 11–18.

Muwonge, Joe Wamala. 1980. "Urban Policy and Patterns of Low-Income Settlement in Nairobi, Kenya." *Population and Development Review* 6 (4): 595–613.

Narayan, K. M. Venkat, Desmond Williams, Edward W Gregg, and Catherine C Cowie. 2011. *Diabetes Public Health*. Oxford, UK: Oxford University Press.

NASCOP (National AIDS and STI Control Programme). 2014. *Kenya HIV Estimates 2014*. Nairobi, Kenya: NASCOP.

Ndetei, David M., Lincoln I. Khasakhala, Mary W. Kuria, Victoria N. Mutiso, Francisca A. Ongecha-Owuor, and Donald A. Kokonya. 2009. "The Prevalence of Mental Disorders in Adults in Different Level General Medical Facilities in Kenya: A Cross-Sectional Study." *Annals of General Psychiatry* 8: 1.

Ndetei, David M, Lincoln I. Khasakhala, Victoria Mutiso, and Anne W. Mbwayo. 2010. "Suicidality and Depression among Adult Patients Admitted in General Medical Facilities in Kenya." *Annals of General Psychiatry* 9: 7.

Needham, Belinda, and Terrence D Hill. 2010. "Do Gender Differences in Mental Health Contribute to Gender Differences in Physical Health?" *Social Science & Medicine* 71 (8): 1472–79.

Nestle, Marion. 2013. *Food Politics: How the Food Industry Influences Nutrition and Health*. Berkeley: University of California Press. 2nd ed.

———. 2015. *Soda Politics: Taking on Big Soda (and Winning)*. Oxford, UK: Oxford University Press.

Nguyen, Vinh-Kim, and Karine Peschard. 2003. "Anthropology, Inequality, and Disease: A Review." *Annual Review of Anthropology* 32: 447–74.

Nichter, Mark. 2001. "The Political Ecology of Health in India: Indigestion as Sign and Symptom of Defective Modernization." In *Healing Powers and Modernity: Traditional Medicine, Shamanism, and Science in Asian Societies*, edited by Linda H. Connor and Geoffrey Samuel, 85–108. Westport, CT: Bergin and Garvey.

———. 2008. *Global Health: Why Cultural Perceptions, Social Representations, and Biopolitics Matter*. Tucson: University of Arizona Press.

Niessen, Louis W., Diwakar Mohan, Jonathan K. Akuoku, Andrew J. Mirelman, Sayem Ahmed, Tracey P. Koehlmoos, Antonio Trujillo, Jahangir Khan, and David H. Peters. 2018. "Tackling Socioeconomic Inequalities and Non-Communicable Diseases in Low-Income and Middle-Income Countries under the Sustainable Development Agenda." *Lancet* 6736 (18): 1–11.

Nordstrom, Carolyn. 2009. "Fault Lines." In *Global Health in Times of Violence*, edited by Barbara Rylko-Bauer, Linda Whiteford, and Paul Farmer, 63–87. Santa Fe, NM: School for Advanced Research Press.

Norris, Shane A., Clive Osmond, Denise Gigante, Chris W. Kuzawa, Lakshmy Ramakrishnan, Nanette R. Lee, Manual Ramirez-Zea, et al. 2012. "Size at Birth, Weight Gain in Infancy and Childhood, and Adult Diabetes Risk in Five Low- or Middle-Income Country Birth Cohorts." *Diabetes Care* 35 (1): 72–79.

Nugent, Rachel, Melanie Y. Bertram, Stephen Jan, Louis W. Niessen, Franco Sassi, Dean T. Jamison, Eduardo González Pier, and Robert Beaglehole. 2018. "Investing in Non-Communicable Disease Prevention and Management to Advance the Sustainable Development Goals." *Lancet* 6736 (18): 1–7.

Nyirenda, Makandwe, Marie Louise Newell, Joseph Mugisha, Portia C. Mutevedzi, Janet Seeley, Francien Scholten, and Paul Kowal. 2013. "Health, Wellbeing, and Disability among Older People Infected or Affected by HIV in Uganda and South Africa." *Global Health Action* 6: 19201.

Nyirenda, Makandwe, Somnath Chatterji, Jane Falkingham, Portia Mutevedzi, Victoria Hosegood, Maria Evandrou, Paul Kowal, and Marie-louise Newell. 2012. "An Investigation of Factors Associated with the Health and Well-Being of HIV-Infected or HIV-Affected Older People in Rural South Africa." *BMC Public Health* 12 (1): 259.

Ochs, Eleanor, and Lisa Capps. 2001. *Living Narrative: Creating Lives in Everyday Storytelling*. Cambridge, MA: Harvard University Press.

Ogaro, Thomas D., W. Githui, Gideon Kikuvi, J. Okari, V. Asiko, E. Wangui, Annemarie Jordaan, Paul D. Van Helden, Elizabeth Maria Streicher, and Thomas C. Victor. 2012. "Diversity of Mycobacterium Tuberculosis Strains in Nairobi, Kenya." *African Journal of Health Sciences* 20: 82–90.

Oni, Tolu, and Nigel Unwin. 2015. "Why the Communicable/Non-Communicable Disease Dichotomy Is Problematic for Public Health Control Strategies: Implications of Multimorbidity for Health Systems in an Era of Health Transition." *International Health* 7 (6): 390–99.

Opwora, Antony, Evelyn Waweru, Mitsuru Toda, Abdisalan Noor, Tansy Edwards, Greg Fegan, Sassy Molyneux, and Catherine Goodman. 2015. "Implementation of Patient Charges at Primary Care Facilities in Kenya: Implications of Low Adherence to User Fee Policy for Users and Facility Revenue." *Health Policy and Planning* 30 (4): 508–17.

Oti, Samuel O., Steven J. M. van de Vijver, Charles Agyemang, and Catherine Kyobutungi. 2013. "The Magnitude of Diabetes and Its Association with Obesity in the Slums of Nairobi, Kenya: Results from a Cross-Sectional Survey." *Tropical Medicine & International Health* 18 (12): 1520–30.

Oxlade, Olivia, and Megan Murray. 2012. "Tuberculosis and Poverty: Why Are the Poor at Greater Risk in India?" *PLoS ONE* 7 (11): 1–8.

Pablos-Méndez, Ariel, Jan Blustein, and Charles A. Knirsch. 1997. "The Role of Diabetes Mellitus in the Higher Prevalence of Tuberculosis among Hispanics." *American Journal of Public Health* 87: 574–79.

Padmanathan, Prianka, and Mary DeSilva. 2013. "The Acceptability and Feasibility of Task-sharing for Mental Healthcare in Low- and Middle-Income Countries: A Systematic Review." *Social Science & Medicine* 97: 82–86.

Page-Reeves, Janet, Joshua Niforatos, Shiraz Mishra, Lidia Regino, Andrew Gingrich, and Robert Bulten. 2013. "Health Disparity and Structural Violence: How Fear Undermines Health among Immigrants at Risk for Diabetes." *Journal of Health Disparities Research and Practice* 6 (2): 30–47.

Parsons, Talcott. 1951. *The Social System.* Glencoe, IL: The Free Press.

Pastakia, Sonak D., Shamim M. Ali, Jemima H. Kamano, Constantine O. Akwanalo, Samson K. Ndege, Victor L. Buckwalter, Rajesh Vedanthan, and Gerald S. Bloomfield. 2013. "Screening for Diabetes and Hypertension in a Rural Low Income Setting in Western Kenya Utilizing Home-Based and Community-Based Strategies." *Globalization and Health* 9: 21.

Patel, Raj. 2012. *Stuffed and Starved: The Hidden Battle for the World Food System.* New York: Melville House.

Patel, Vikram, Fungisai Gwanzura, Essie Simunyu, K. S. Lloyd, Anthony Mann. 1995a. "The phenomenology and explanatory models of common mental disorder: a study in primary care in Harare, Zimbabwe." Psychological Med 25, 1191–1200.

Patel, Vikram, Essie Simunyu, Fungisai Gwanzura. 1995b. "Kufungisisa (Thinking Too Much): A Shona Idiom for Non-psychotic Mental Illness." *Central African Journal of Medicine* 41, 209–215.

Patel, Vikram, Helen A. Weiss, Neerja Chowdhary, Smita Naik, Sulochana Pednekar, Sudipto Chatterjee, Bhargav Bhat, et al. 2011. "Lay Health Worker Led Intervention for Depressive and Anxiety Disorders in India: Impact on Clinical and Disability Outcomes over 12 Months." *British Journal of Psychiatry* 199 (6): 459–66.

Patel, Vikram, Jerson Pereira, Livia Coutinho, Romaldina Fernandes, Jefferson Fernandes, and Anthony Mann. 1998. "Poverty, Psychological Disorder and Disability in Primary Care Attenders in Goa, India." *British Journal of Psychiatry* 172: 533–36.

Patel, Vikram, Merlyn Rodrigues, and Nandita DeSouza. 2002. "Gender, Poverty, and Postnatal Depression: A Study of Mothers in Goa, India." *American Journal of Psychiatry* 159 (1): 43–47.

Peden, Margie, Kara S. McGee, and Gyanendra Sharma. 2002. *The Injury Chart Book: A Graphical Overview of the Global Burden of Injuries.* Geneva, Switzerland: WHO.

Peer, Nasheeta, Krisela Steyn, Carl Lombard, Estelle V. Lambert, Bavanisha Vythilingum, and Naomi S. Levitt. 2012. "Rising Diabetes Prevalence among Urban-Dwelling Black South Africans." *PLoS ONE* 7 (9): e43336.

Peltzer, Karl. 2009. "Traditional Health Practitioners in South Africa." *Lancet* 374 (9694): 956–57.

Petersen, Inge, Crick Lund, Arvin Bhana, and Alan J. Flisher. 2012. "A Task Shifting Approach to Primary Mental Health Care for Adults in South Africa: Human Resource Requirements and Costs for Rural Settings." *Health Policy and Planning* 27 (1): 42–51.

Petrak, Frank, Harold Baumeister, Timothy C. Skinner, Alex Brown, and Richard I. G. Holt. 2015. "Depression and Diabetes: Treatment and Health-Care Delivery." *Lancet* 3: 472–85.

Phelan, Jo C., Bruce G. Link, Ana Diez-Roux, Ichiro Kawachi, and Bruce Levin. 2004. "'Fundamental Causes' of Social Inequalities in Mortality: A Test of the Theory." *Journal of Health and Social Behavior* 45(3), 265–85.

Phelan, Jo C., Bruce G. Link, and Parisa Tehranifar. 2010. "Social Conditions as Fundamental Causes of Health Inequalities: Theory, Evidence, and Policy Implications." *Journal of Health and Social Behavior* 51 (Suppl.): S28–40.

Pickett, Kate E., Shona Kelly, Eric Brunner, Tim Lobstein, and Richard G. Wilkinson. 2005. "Wider Income Gaps, Wider Waistbands? An Ecological Study of Obesity and Income Inequality." *Journal of Epidemiology and Community Health* 59: 670–74.

Ponce-De-Leon, Alfredo, de Lordes Garcia-Garcia, Ma Cecilia Garcia-Sancho, Francisco J. Gomez-Perez, Jose Luis Valdespino-Gomez, Gustavo Olaiz-Fernandez, Rosalba Rojas, et al. 2004. "Tuberculosis and Diabetes in Southern Mexico." *Diabetes Care* 27: 1584–90.

Poongothai, Subramani, Rajendra Pradeepa, Anbhazhagan Ganesan, and Viswanathan Mohan. 2009. "Prevalence of Depression in a Large Urban South Indian Population—The Chennai Urban Rural Epidemiology Study (Cures—70)." *PLoS ONE* 4(9): e7185.

Popkin, Barry M. 2006. "Global Nutrition Dynamics: The World Is Shifting Rapidly toward a Diet Linked with Noncommunicable Diseases." *American Journal of Clinical Nutrition* 84 (2): 289–98.

——. 2015. "Nutrition Transition and the Global Diabetes Epidemic." *Current Diabetes Reports* 15 (9): 64.

Popkin, Barry M., and Corinna Hawkes. 2015. "Sweetening of the Global Diet, Particularly Beverages: Patterns, Trends, and Policy Responses." *Lancet Diabetes & Endocrinology* 4 (2): 174–86.

Popkin, Barry M., Linda S. Adair, and Shu Wen Ng. 2012. "Global Nutrition Transition and the Pandemic of Obesity in Developing Countries." *Nutrition Reviews* 70 (1): 3–21.

Posel, Dorrit, and Michael Rogan. 2012. "Gendered Trends in Poverty in the Post-Apartheid Period, 1997–2006." *Development Southern Africa* 29 (1): 97–113.

Pouwer, Frans, Nina Kupper, and Marcel C Adriaanse. 2010. "Does Emotional Stress Cause Type 2 Diabetes Mellitus? A Review from the European Depression in Diabetes (EDID) Research Consortium." *Discovery Medicine* 9 (45): 112–18.

Pratt, Laura A., and Debra J. Brody. 2014. "Depression in the U.S. Household Population, 2009–2012." NCHS Data Brief 172 (December): 1–8.

Preiss, Kymberlie, Leah Brennan, and David Clarke. 2013. "A Systematic Review of Variables Associated with the Relationship between Obesity and Depression." *Obesity Reviews* 14: 906–18.

Prince, Martin, Vikram Patel, Shekhar Saxena, Mario Maj, Joanna Maselko, Michael R. Phillips, and Atif Rahman. 2007. "No Health without Mental Health." *Lancet* 370: 859–77.

Quigley, Fran, 2009. *Walking Together, Walking Far: How a U.S. and African Medical School Partnership Is Winning the Fight against HIV/AIDS*. Indianapolis: University of Indiana Press.

Radin, Paul. 1983. *Crashing Thunder: The Autobiography of an American Indian*. Lincoln: University of Nebraska Press. Originally published 1926.

Radloff, Lenore Sawyer. 1977. "The CES-D Scale." *Applied Psychological Measurement* 1 (3): 385–401.

Rahman, Atif, Abid Malik, Siham Sikander, Christopher Roberts, and Francis Creed. 2008a. "Cognitive Behaviour Therapy-Based Intervention by Community Health Workers for Mothers with Depression and Their Infants in Rural Pakistan: A Cluster-Randomised Controlled Trial." *Lancet* 372 (9642): 902–9.

Rahman, Atif, Vikram Patel, Joanna Maselko, and Betty Kirkwood. 2008b. "The Neglected 'M' in MCH Programmes—Why Mental Health of Mothers Is Important for Child Nutrition." *Tropical Medicine & International Health* 13 (4): 579–83.

Remais, Justin V., Guang Zeng, Guangwei Li, Lulu Tian, and Michael M. Engelgau. 2013. "Convergence of Non-Communicable and Infectious Diseases in Low- and Middle-Income Countries." *International Journal of Epidemiology* 42 (1): 221–27.

Renn, Brenna N., Leilani Feliciano, and Daniel L. Segal. 2011. "The Bidirectional Relationship of Depression and Diabetes: A Systematic Review." *Clinical Psychology Review* 31 (8): 1239–46.

Rhodes, Tim, Merrill Singer, Philippe Bourgois, Samuel R. Friedman, and Steffanie A. Strathdee. 2005. "The Social Structural Production of HIV Risk among Injecting Drug Users." *Social Science & Medicine* 61: 1026–44.

Rich, Stephen S. 2016. "Diabetes: Still a Geneticist's Nightmare." *Nature* 536 (7614): 37–38.

Richter, Linda M., Shane A. Norris, John Pettifor, Derek Yach, and Noel Cameron. 2007. "Cohort Profile: Mandela's Children: The 1990 Birth to Twenty Study in South Africa." *International Journal of Epidemiology* 36: 504–11.

Riza, Anca Lelia, Fiona Pearson, Cesar Ugarte-Gil, Bachti Alisjahbana, Steven van de Vijver, Nicolae M Panduru, Philip C Hill, et al. 2014. "Clinical Management of Concurrent Diabetes and Tuberculosis and the Implications for Patient Services." *Lancet Diabetes & Endocrinology* 2 (9): 740–53.

Rock, Melanie. 2003. "Sweet Blood and Social Suffering: Rethinking Cause-Effect Relationships in Diabetes, Distress, and Duress." *Medical Anthropology* 22 (2): 131–74.

———. 2005. "Classifying Diabetes; or, Commensurating Bodies of Unequal Experience." *Public Culture* 17 (3): 467–86.

Rose, Geoffrey. 1981. "Strategy of Prevention: Lessons from Cardiovascular Disease." *BMJ* 282: 1847–51.

———. 1985. "Sick Individuals and Sick Populations." *International Journal of Epidemiology* 30: 427–32.

Rosenberg, Charles E. 1992. *Explaining Epidemics and Other Studies in the History of Medicine*. New York: Cambridge University Press.

Ruel-Bergeron, Julie C., Gretchen A. Stevens, Jonathan D. Sugimoto, Franz F. Roos, Majid Ezzati, Robert E. Black, and Klaus Kraemer. 2015. "Global Update and Trends of Hidden Hunger, 1995–2011: The Hidden Hunger Index." *PLoS One* 10 (12): 1–13.

Sapolsky, Robert. 2004. *Why Zebras Don't Get Ulcers: The Acclaimed Guide to Stress, Stress-Related Diseases, and Coping*. New York: W. H. Freeman and Company. 3rd ed.

Sassi, Franco, Annalisa Belloni, Andrew J. Mirelman, Marc Suhrcke, Alastair Thomas, Nisreen Salti, Sukumar Vellakkal, Chonlathan Visaruthvong, Barry M. Popkin, and Rachel Nugent. 2018. "Equity Impacts of Price Policies to Promote Healthy Behaviours." *Lancet* 391 (10134): 2059–70.

Schabert, Jasmin, Jessica L. Browne, Kylie Mosely, and Jane Speight. 2013. "Social Stigma in Diabetes: A Framework to Understand a Growing Problem for an Increasing Epidemic." *Patient* 6 (1): 1–10.

Scheder, Jo C. 1988. "A Sickly-Sweet Harvest: Farmworker Diabetes and Social Equality." *Medical Anthropology Quarterly* 2 (3): 251–77.

Scheper-Hughes, Nancy. 1989. "Death without Weeping: Has Poverty Ravaged Mother Love in the Shantytowns of Brazil?" *The Human Strategy* 10: 8–16.

———. 1992. *Death without Weeping: The Violence of Everyday Life in Brazil*. Berkeley: University of California Press.

Schneider, Mary L., and Colleen F. Moore. 2000. "Effects of Prenatal Stress on Development: A Nonhuman Primate Model." In *The Effects of Early Adversity on Neurobehavioral Development: The Minnesota Symposia on Child Psychology*, vol. 31, edited by Charles A. Nelson, 201–44. Mahwah, NJ.: Lawrence Erlbaum Associates.

Schoenberg, Nancy E., Elaine M. Drew, Eleanor Palo Stoller, and Cary S. Kart. 2005. "Situating Stress: Lessons from Lay Discourses on Diabetes." *Medical Anthropology Quarterly* 19 (2): 171–93.

Scholten, Franciene, Joseph Mugisha, Janet Seeley, Eugene Kinyanda, Susan Naku-bukwa, Paul Kowal, Nirmala Naidoo, Ties Boerma, Somnath Chatterji, and Heiner Grosskurth. 2011. "Health and Functional Status among Older People with HIV/AIDS in Uganda." *BMC Public Health* 11 (1): 886.

Schulz, Amy J., and Leith Mullings. 2006. *Gender, Race, Class & Health: Intersectional Approaches*. New York: Jossey-Bass.

Seeberg, Jens, and Lotte Meinert. 2015. "Can Epidemics Be Noncommunicable? Reflections on the Spread of 'Noncommunicable' Diseases." *Medicine Anthropology Theory* 2: 54–71.

Seedat, Mohamed, Ashley Van Niekerk, Rachel Jewkes, Shahnaaz Suffla, and Kopano Ratele. 2009. "Violence and Injuries in South Africa: Prioritising an Agenda for Prevention." *Lancet* 374: 1011–22.

Seligman, Rebecca. 2010. "The Unmaking and Making of Self: Embodied Suffering and Mind–Body Healing in Brazilian Candomblé." *Ethos* 38 (3): 297–320.

Seligman, Rebecca, Emily Mendenhall, Maria D. Valdovinos, Alicia Fernandez, and Elizabeth A. Jacobs. 2015. "Self-Care and Subjectivity among Mexican Diabetes Patients in the United States." *Medical Anthropology Quarterly* 29 (1): 61–79.

Sherr, Lorraine, Claudine Clucas, Richard Harding, Elissa Sibley, and Jose Catalan. 2011. "HIV and Depression—A Systematic Review of Interventions." *Psychology, Health & Medicine* 16 (5): 493–527.

Shiffman, Jeremy. 2008. "Has Donor Prioritization of HIV/AIDS Displaced Aid for Other Health Issues?" *Health Policy and Planning* 23 (2): 95–100.

Shisana, Olive, Thomas Rehle, Leickness Simbayi, Demetre Labadarios, Sean Jooste, Alicia Davids, Shandir Ramlagan, et al. 2012. *South African National HIV Prevalence, Incidence and Behaviour Survey, 2012*. Pretoria, South Africa: Human Sciences Research Council.

Singer, Merrill. 1994. "Aids and the Health Crisis of the U.S. Urban Poor: The Perspective of Critical Medical Anthropology." *Social Science & Medicine* 39 (7): 931–48.

——. 1996. "A Dose of Drugs, a Touch of Violence, a Case of AIDS: Conceptualizing the SAVA Syndemic." *Free Inquiry in Creative Sociology* 24 (2): 99–110.

——. 2003. "Syndemics and Public Health: Reconceptualizing Disease in Bio-Social Context." *Medical Anthropology Quarterly* 17 (4): 423–41.

——. 2009. *Introduction to Syndemics: A Systems Approach to Public and Community Health*. San Francisco: Jossey-Bass.

Singer, Merrill, Nicola Bulled, Bayla Ostrach, and Emily Mendenhall. 2017. "Syndemics and the Biosocial Conception of Health." *Lancet* 389: 941–50.

Singer, Merrill, Pamela I. Erickson, Louise Badiane, Rosemary Diaz, Dugeidy Ortiz, Traci Abraham, and Anna Marie. 2006. "Syndemics, Sex and the City: Understanding Sexually Transmitted Diseases in Social and Cultural Context." *Social Science & Medicine* 63: 2010–21.

Singer, Merrill, and Scott Clair. 2003. "Syndemics and Public Health: Reconceptualizing Disease in Bio-Social Context." *Medical Anthropology Quarterly* 17 (4): 423–41.

Singer, Merrill, Tom Stopka, Cara Siano, Kristen Springer, George Barton, Kaveh Khoshnood, April Gorry De Puga, and Robert Heimer. 2000. "The Social Geography of AIDS and Hepatitis Risk: Qualitative Approaches for Assessing Local Differences in Sterile-Syringe Access among Injection Drug Users." *American Journal of Public Health* 90 (7): 1049–56.

Singla, Daisy R., Elias Kumbakumba, and Frances E. Aboud. 2015. "Effects of a Parenting Intervention to Address Maternal Psychological Wellbeing and Child Development and Growth in Rural Uganda: A Community-Based, Cluster-Randomised Trial." *Lancet Global Health* 3 (8): e458–69.

Smith-Morris, Carolyn. 2008. *Diabetes among the Pima: Stories of Survival*. Tucson: University of Arizona Press.

———. 2010. "The Chronicity of Life, the Acuteness of Diagnosis." In *Chronic Conditions, Fluid States: Chronicity and the Anthropology of Illness*, edited by Lenore Manderson and Carolyn Smith-Morris, 21–37. New Brunswick, NJ: Rutgers University Press.

Snell-Rood, Claire. 2015. "Marital Distress and the Failure to Eat: The Expressive Dimensions of Feeding, Eating, and Self-Care in Urban South Asia." *Medical Anthropology Quarterly* 29 (3): 316–33.

Snoek, Frank J., Marijke A. Bremmer, and Norbert Hermanns. 2015. "Constructs of Depression and Distress in Diabetes: Time for an Appraisal." *Lancet* 3: 450–60.

Soler, J., V. Perez-Sola, D. Puigdemont, J. Perez-Blanco, M. Figueres, and E. Alvarez. 1997. "Validation Study of the Center for Epidemiological Studies—Depression of a Spanish Population of Patients with Affective Disorders." *Actas Luso-Espanolas de Neurologia, Psiquiatria y Ciencias Afines* 25 (4): 243–49.

Solomon, Harris. 2016. *Metabolic Living: Food, Fat, and the Absorption of Illness in India*. Durham, NC: Duke University Press.

Stall, Ron, Mark Friedman, and Joseph Catania. 2008. "Interacting Epidemics and Gay Men's Health: A Theory of Syndemic Production among Urban Gay Men." In *Unequal Opportunity: Health Disparities Affecting Gay and Bisexual Men in the United States*, edited by Richard J. Wolitski, Ron Stall, and Ronald O. Valdiserri. Oxford, UK: Oxford University Press.

Steel, Zachary, Claire Marnane, Changiz Iranpour, Tien Chey, John W. Jackson, Vikram Patel, and Derrick Silove. 2014. "The Global Prevalence of Common Mental Disorders: A Systematic Review and Meta-Analysis 1980–2013." *International Journal of Epidemiology* 43 (2): 476–93.

Stein, Dan J., Soraya Seedat, Allen Herman, Hashim Moomal, Steven G. Heeringa, Ronald C. Kessler, and David R. Williams. 2008. "Lifetime Prevalence of Psychiatric Disorders in South Africa." *British Journal of Psychiatry* 192 (2): 112–17.

Stringhini, Silvia, Cristian Carmeli, Markus Jokela, Mauricio Avendaño, Peter Muennig, Florence Guida, Fulvio Ricceri, et al. 2017. "Socioeconomic Status and the 25x25 Risk Factors as Determinants of Premature Mortality: A Multicohort Study and Meta-Analysis of 1.7 Million Men and Women." *Lancet* 6736 (16): 7–9.

Stuckler, David, and Marion Nestle. 2012. "Big Food, Food Systems, and Global Health." *PLoS Medicine* 9 (6): 7.

Stuckler, David, and Sanjay Basu. 2013. *The Body Economic: Why Austerity Kills*. New York: Basic Books.

Swart, Elizabeth. 2011. "Strategies for Coping with Gender-Based Violence: A Study of Young Women In Kibera." Master's Thesis, University of Central Florida.

Talbot, France, and Arie Nouwen. 2000. "A Review of the Relationship between Depression and Diabetes in Adults: Is There a Link?" *Diabetes Care* 23 (10): 1556–62.

Taubes, Gary. 2011. *Why We Get Fat and What to Do about It.* New York: Anchor Books.

——. 2017. *The Case against Sugar.* New York: Anchor Books.

Thayer, Zaneta M., and Amy L. Non. 2015. "Anthropology Meets Epigenetics: Current and Future Directions." *American Anthropologist* 117 (4): 722–35.

Thayer, Zaneta, Celestina Barbosa-Leiker Michael, Lonnie Nelson, Dedra Buchwald, and Spero Manson. 2016. "Early Life Trauma, Post-Traumatic Stress Disorder, and Allostatic Load in a Sample of American Indian Adults." *American Journal of Human Biology* 29 (3): 1–10.

Thayer, Zaneta M., and Christopher W. Kuzawa. 2011. "Biological Memories of Past Environments: Epigenetic Pathways to Health Disparities." *Epigenetics* 6 (7): 798–803.

Tregenna, Fiona, and Mfanafuthi Tsela. 2012. "Inequality in South Africa: The Distribution of Income, Expenditure and Earnings." *Development Southern Africa* 29 (1): 35–61.

Tsai, Alexander C., Emily Mendenhall, James Trostle, and Ichiro Kawachi. 2017. "Co-Occurring Epidemics, Syndemics, and Population Health." *Lancet* 389: 978–82.

Turner, Victor. 1969. *The Ritual Process: Structure and Anti-Structure.* Chicago: Aldine.

Vellakkal, Sukumar, Christopher Millett, Sanjay Basu, Zaky Khan, Amina Aitsi-Selmi, David Stuckler, and Shah Ebrahim. 2014. "Are Estimates of Socioeconomic Inequalities in Chronic Disease Artefactually Narrowed by Self-Reported Measures of Prevalence in Low-Income and Middle-Income Countries? Findings from the WHO-SAGE Survey." *Journal of Epidemiology and Community Health* 69 (3): 218–25.

Vellakkal, Sukumar, S. V. Subramanian, Christopher Millett, Sanjay Basu, David Stuckler, and Shah Ebrahim. 2013. "Socioeconomic Inequalities in Non-Communicable Diseases Prevalence in India: Disparities between Self-Reported Diagnoses and Standardized Measures." *PLoS One* 8 (7): e68219.

Walker, Rebekah J., Mulugeta Gebregziabher, Bonnie Martin-Harris, and Leonard E. Egede. 2015. "Quantifying Direct Effects of Social Determinants of Health on Glycemic Control in Adults with Type 2 Diabetes." *Diabetes Technology & Therapeutics* 17 (2): 80–87.

Walker, Renee E., Christopher R. Keane, and Jessica G. Burke. 2010. "Disparities and Access to Healthy Food in the United States: A Review of Food Deserts Literature." *Health & Place* 16: 876–84.

Weaver, Lesley Jo. 2016. "Transactions in Suffering: Mothers, Daughters, and Chronic Disease Comorbidities in New Delhi, India." *Medical Anthropology Quarterly* 30 (4): 498–514.

——. 2017. "Tension Among Women in North India: An Idiom of Distress and a Cultural Syndrome." *Culture, Medicine, and Psychiatry* 41 (1): 35–55.

Weaver, Lesley Jo, Carol M. Worthman, Jason A. DeCaro, and S. V. Madhu. 2015. "The Signs of Stress: Embodiments of Biosocial Stress among Type 2 Diabetic Women in New Delhi, India." *Social Science & Medicine* 131: 122–30.

Weaver, Lesley Jo, and Craig Hadley. 2011. "Social Pathways in the Comorbidity between Type 2 Diabetes and Mental Health Concerns in a Pilot Study of Urban Middle- and Upper-Class Indian Women." *Ethos* 39 (2): 211–25.

Weaver, Lesley Jo, and Emily Mendenhall. 2014. "Applying Syndemics and Chronicity: Interpretations from Studies of Poverty, Depression, and Diabetes." *Medical Anthropology* 33 (2): 92–108.

Weller, Susan C., Roberta D. Baer, Javier Garcia De Alba Garcia, and Ana L. Salcedo Rocha. 2008. "Susto and Nervios: Expressions for Stress and Depression." *Culture, Medicine, and Psychiatry* 32 (3): 406–20.

Werfalli, Mahmoud, Peter Raubenheimer, Mark Engel, Nasheeta Peer, Sebastiana Kalula, Andre P. Kengne, and Naomi S. Levitt. 2015. "Effectiveness of Community-Based Peer-Led Diabetes Self-Management Programmes (COMP-DSMP) for Improving Clinical Outcomes and Quality of Life of Adults with Diabetes in Primary Care Settings in Low and Middle-Income Countries (LMIC): A Systematic Review and Meta-Analysis." *BMJ Open* 5 (7): e007635.

WHO (World Health Organization). 2007. *Everybody's Business: Strengthening Health Systems to Improve Health Outcomes: WHO's Framework for Action*. Geneva, Switzerland: WHO.

———. 2008. *Task Shifting: Rational Redistribution of Tasks among Health Workforce Teams: Global Recommendations and Guidelines*. Geneva, Switzerland: WHO.

———. 2014. *Global Tuberculosis Report 2014*. Geneva, Switzerland: WHO.

Wiedman, Dennis. 2012. "Native American Embodiment of the Chronicities of Modernity: Reservation Food, Diabetes, and the Metabolic Syndrome among the Kiowa, Comanche, and Apache." *Medical Anthropology Quarterly* 26 (4): 595–612.

Willen, Sarah S. 2007. "Toward a Critical Phenomenology of 'Illegality': State Power, Criminalization, and Abjectivity among Undocumented Migrant Workers in Tel Aviv, Israel." *International Migration* 45 (3): 8–38.

Willen, Sarah S., Michael Knipper, Cesar Abadia-Barrero, and Nadav Davidovitch. 2017. "Syndemic Vulnerability and the Right to Health." *Lancet* 389: 964–77.

Wood, Kate, and Helen Lambert. 2008. "Coded Talk, Scripted Omissions: The Micropolitics of AIDS Talk in South Africa." *Medical Anthropology Quarterly* 22 (3): 213–33.

Wynne, Katie, Sarah Stanley, Barbara McGowan, and Steve Bloom. 2005. "Appetite Control." *The Journal of Endocrinology* 184 (2): 291–318.

Yach, Derek, David Stuckler, and Kelly D Brownell. 2006. "Epidemiologic and Economic Consequences of the Global Epidemics of Obesity and Diabetes." *Nature Medicine* 12 (1): 62–66.

Yates-Doerr, Emily. 2015. *The Weight of Obesity: Hunger and Global Health in Postwar Guatemala*. Berkeley: University of California Press.

Yuen, Courtney M., Herman O. Weyenga, Andrea A. Kim, Timothy Malika, Hellen Muttai, Abraham Katana, Lucy Nganga, Kevin P. Cain, and Kevin M. De Cock. 2014. "Comparison of Trends in Tuberculosis Incidence among Adults Living with HIV and Adults without HIV—Kenya, 1998–2012." *PLoS One* 9 (6): 1–7.

Zabetian, Azadeh, Isabelle M. Sanchez, K. M. Venkat Narayan, Christopher K. Hwang, and Mohammed K. Ali. 2014. "Global Rural Diabetes Prevalence: A Systematic

Review and Meta-Analysis Covering 1990–2012." *Diabetes Research and Clinical Practice* 104 (2): 206–12.

Zimmet, Paul Z. 2017. "Diabetes and Its Drivers: The Largest Epidemic in Human History?" *Clinical Diabetes and Endocrinology* 3 (1): 1–8.

Zuch, Melanie, and Mark Lurie. 2012. "'A Virus and Nothing Else': The Effect of ART on HIV-Related Stigma in Rural South Africa." *AIDS and Behavior* 16 (3): 564–70.

Index

Note: Italicized page numbers followed by an *f* or *t* indicate figures or tables respectively.